Community-Based Integrated Care for Older Adults

Matthew K. McNabney
Editor

Community-Based Integrated Care for Older Adults

A Practical Guide

Springer

Editor
Matthew K. McNabney
Hopkins ElderPlus
Johns Hopkins University
Baltimore, MD, USA

Associate Editors
Judith Baskins
Heath Care Consultant, PACE Project Manager, South Carolina Department of Health and Human Services
Columbia, SC, USA

G. Paul Eleazer
Clinical Innovations
Geriatric Research and Education Center (GRECC)
Salt Lake City VA Medical Center
Salt Lake City, UT, USA

ISBN 978-3-031-05136-4 ISBN 978-3-031-05137-1 (eBook)
https://doi.org/10.1007/978-3-031-05137-1

This Springer imprint is published by the registered company Springer Nature Switzerland AG
The registered company address is: Gewerbestrasse 11, 6330 Cham, Switzerland

Preface

Older adults are a heterogenous group. Many people maintain good health and high functional status well into late life. However, as people age there is an increased likelihood of medical illnesses as well as functional and cognitive impairment. If that were not enough challenge for older adults and their families, there are also social and financial factors that can complicate management and can become overwhelming for people living in the community. This can lead to additional strain on the family network and often leads to placement in long-term care facilities, such as nursing homes and assisted living facilities.

Adequacy of medical care is also an issue for many older adults who live daily lives in a precarious medical state. Typical primary care practices are not adequately designed or funded to provide the intensive care coordination and timely interventions needed to avoid decompensation of chronic medical illnesses and avoidable hospitalizations.

Certainly, nursing homes are sometimes necessary to ensure adequate care and safety. However, there are many circumstances where a comprehensive and coordinated package of services could help to postpone or eliminate the need for placement in a facility. When targeting older adults who are at the greatest need, the care requirements and coordination needs can be quite intense and costly. Funding streams for older adults have largely come from Medicare and Medicaid. These funding sources have mostly led patients and their caregivers to work with primary care providers and specialists until they are unable to maintain themselves in the community and have no choice but to move into a nursing home.

Over the past few decades, there have been a few models of care designed to address those needs and allow older adults to remain in the community. Many start as "waiver programs" to allow for a demonstration of benefit and feasibility. Some programs survive, many do not. An important example of a successful community-based integrated care model is the Program of All-Inclusive Care for the Elderly (PACE).

PACE was started as a demonstration program in the 1980s. Multiple studies have demonstrated its financial impact and benefits to patients and their caregivers. As a result, PACE achieved "permanent provider" status within the Centers for

Medicare and Medicaid (CMS) in 1997. PACE now serves several thousand older adults in the United States who have been certified as eligible for nursing homes but can be managed in the community with a large, well-trained, interdisciplinary team.

This book is a first of its kind. It provides a comprehensive overview of community-based integrated care, with a primary focus on PACE. It is a practical guide, written by those closely involved with PACE, and is intended to walk the reader through the many layers that are required to achieve this level of service coordination. The chapters covering PACE include chapters that review "big picture" topics such as starting a program, policy considerations, and leadership development. There are also individual chapters on the various roles and function of the interdisciplinary team, which is often considered the "secret sauce" of PACE.

We hope this book is helpful to those who are interested in starting a PACE program as well as those who are studying this process to gain expertise in public health policy and finance.

Baltimore, MD, USA Matthew K. McNabney

Contents

Contributors

Hidenori Arai National Center for Geriatrics and Gerontology, Obu, Aichi, Japan

Mary Austin Senior Pathways LLC, Phoenixville, PA, USA

Sarah Babineau Providence ElderPlace, Seattle, WA, USA

Judith Baskins Heath Care Consultant, PACE Project Manager, South Carolina Department of Health and Human Services, Columbia, SC, USA

Shawn Bloom National PACE Association, Alexandria, VA, USA

Janice Braxton Social Work Department, Piedmont Health Senior Care, Burlington, NC, USA

Lori Calkins Nursing/Operations, Providence ElderPlace, Seaside, OR, USA

Ulrike Dapp Research Department, Albertinen-Haus Geriatrics Center, University of Hamburg, Hamburg, Germany

Peter DeGolia McGregor PACE, Cleveland, OH, USA

Susan Disman Providence ElderPlace Washington Providence St. Joseph Health, Seattle, WA, USA

Emily Drennan PACE Organization of Rhode Island, Providence, RI, USA

Kelsey Ellis Providence ElderPlace Washington Providence St. Joseph Health, Seattle, WA, USA

Catherine Eng On Lok Senior Health Services, San Francisco, CA, USA

Department of Medicine and Geriatrics, UCSF School of Medicine, San Francisco, CA, USA

Suzanne Fortune Quality and Patient Safety, Ascension Living HOPE, Wichita, KS, USA

Ellen Garcia Providence ElderPlace Oregon, Portland, OR, USA

Gwen Graddy-Dansby PACE Southeast Michigan, Dearborn, MI, USA

Gwen Graddy PACE Southeast Michigan, Detroit, MI, USA

Kristie Hartig Community Nursing, Midland Care Connection, Inc, Topeka, KS, USA

Réjean Hébert Department of Health Management, Evaluation and Policy, School of Public Health, Université de Montréal, Montréal, QC, Canada

Sean Hennessy Division of Epidemiology, Department of Biostatistics, Epidemiology and Informatics, University of Pennsylvania Perelman School of Medicine, Philadelphia, PA, USA

Heather Hill Social Work Department, Providence ElderPlace, Portland, OR, USA

April Holmes Hopkins ElderPlus, Baltimore, MD, USA

Lisa Jenkins Supportive Care Services, Community LIFE, Pittsburgh, PA, USA

Dana Kennedy Community LIFE, Pittsburgh, PA, USA

Kathryn Dorward King Rochester, NY, USA

Bruce Kinosian Department of Medicine, University of Pennsylvania Perelman School of Medicine, Philadelphia, PA, USA

Catherine Knuth Milliman, Brookfield, WI, USA

Joan Kwiatkowski PACE Organization of Rhode Island, Providence, RI, USA

Becket Lauten Social Work, Providence ElderPlace, Portland, OR, USA

Yunhwan Lee Department of Preventive Medicine and Public Health, Ajou University School of Medicine, Suwon, Gyeonggi Province, South Korea

Matthew K. McNabney Hopkins ElderPlus, Johns Hopkins University, Baltimore, MD, USA

Richard Mueller Mequon, WI, USA

S. Hanlon Newhall Hopkins ElderPlus, Baltimore, MD, USA

Renee Newmuis Hopkins ElderPlus, Baltimore, MD, USA

June Nicholas Hopkins ElderPlus, Baltimore, MD, USA

Victoria Parker PACE Organization of Rhode Island, Providence, RI, USA

James Pezzuti Harrisburg, PA, USA

Cheryl Phillips SNP Alliance, Washington, DC, USA

Anita Pope Rocky Mountain PACE, Colorado Springs, CO, USA

E. J. Rice Hopkins ElderPlus, Johns Hopkins University, Baltimore, MD, USA

Ashley Souza Neighborhood PACE, East Boston, MA, USA

Deny Stiassny Hopkins ElderPlus, Baltimore, MD, USA

David Wensel TRU Community Care, Lafayette, CO, USA

Part I
Community-Based Integrated Care

Chapter 1
The International Perspective on Community-Based Integrated Care

Yunhwan Lee, Hidenori Arai, Ulrike Dapp, and Réjean Hébert

Introduction

Throughout the world, three factors are driving the development of innovative ways of delivering care to older people in the community: (1) the magnitude of population aging, (2) the complex health and long-term care needs of older adults, and (3) the fragmented services and uncoordinated delivery that not only fail to meet older people's changing care needs but also result in the rising costs of care. The aging world population is increasingly portrayed as "aging of the aged," where the oldest old, aged 80 years or older, are the fastest-growing segment of the older population. Longer years of life are often accompanied by multiple comorbidities and functional disability, sharply increasing demands for health and long-term care. The societal burden of care is increasing, with a disproportionately large portion of older people receiving formal and informal care. The current health care system, which is

---

Y. Lee (✉)
Department of Preventive Medicine and Public Health, Ajou University School of Medicine, Suwon, Gyeonggi Province, South Korea
e mail: yhlee@ajou.ac.kr

H. Arai
National Center for Geriatrics and Gerontology, Obu, Aichi, Japan
e-mail: harai@ncgg.go.jp

U. Dapp
Research Department, Albertinen-Haus Geriatrics Center, University of Hamburg, Hamburg, Germany
e-mail: Ulrike.dapp@albertinen.de

R. Hébert
Department of Health Management, Evaluation and Policy, School of Public Health, Université de Montréal, Montréal, QC, Canada
e-mail: Rejean.Hebert@UMontreal.ca

M. K. McNabney (ed.), *Community-Based Integrated Care for Older Adults*,
https://doi.org/10.1007/978-3-031-05137-1_1

heavily biased toward providing acute care, is not well suited to attend to the difficulties facing older adults, especially those who are frail and functionally impaired. With rising costs of care in institutions, interest has focused on providing services in the home and community. However, organizations and services are often fragmented and the delivery poorly coordinated, generating confusion and dismay as older adults and their families navigate through the maze of different services available in their community.

Community-based integrated care has come to the forefront as a promising approach to mitigating the shortfalls of the current system in providing care to older people with complex needs. Two key concepts underlie community-based integrated care [1].

This includes *community-based care*, also referred to as community care, care in the community, and home and community-based services. It is predicated on the preference of older people to receive care where they live, or what is called "aging in place." Care and support organized at the local and regional levels, reflecting the beliefs and values of the community and drawing on its resources, are more capable of providing services that are aligned to the individual's needs. Shifting the emphasis of care to community settings can reduce the cost of unnecessary admissions to hospitals and nursing homes.

The other concept is *integrated care*, which has various definitions and approaches and aims to effectively coordinate the delivery of a set of comprehensive services according to a person's needs. Integration can occur at the macro (system), meso (organizational and professional), and micro (clinical) levels [2]. Integration may also vary in degree or intensity as linkages, coordination, and full integration [3]. Care arrangements likely involve both vertical (across primary, secondary, and tertiary levels of care, including transitions from hospital to community-based services) and horizontal (between health care, long-term care, and social services) integration [4]. More recently, "person-centered care" has been advocated as a core component of integrated care, in which the person's values and voices are incorporated into the shared decision-making for individualized planning and organizing of services. Integrated care within the health care system or between health and social care appears to increase access to services and perceived quality of care and enhance patient satisfaction [5]. Evidence on cost-savings of integrated care is, however, limited.

Over the years, innovative approaches to providing community-based integrated care to older adults have emerged across the world. Although the way services are developed, organized, delivered, and managed has been strongly influenced by individual countries' social and cultural values, and their health and social care systems, common features of successful models have been identified [6, 7]. At the service and organizational levels, strategies used to achieve the adoption of an integrated care system include comprehensive geriatric assessment; care planning by interdisciplinary teams; case or care management; a single point of entry; coordination of care; integrated housing, support, and care; integration of financing mechanisms;

and quality improvement. In community-based models, which target high-risk populations, especially frail older people, success depends on the active involvement of physicians in managing care; participation of multidisciplinary teams, which include geriatricians; cooperation across care providers in a continuum of care; and care coordination across various community-based and institutional services [8]. It should, however, be noted that although diverse sets of initiatives on integrated care in the community have been implemented, most have not advanced beyond short-term demonstrations to become a part of mainstream services. Failure to consider costs for start-up, service funding, and staff and support systems have hindered not only the implementation but also the maintenance and replication of many promising models [3].

In this chapter, we will consider the experience of four countries in developing community-based integrated care for older people. Each country presents different approaches to coordinating care for older adults to help them continue to live in their communities. The issues and challenges faced in bringing care "home" are discussed.

Canada[1]

Canada is a confederation of ten provinces and three territories. The health care system in Canada was developed in the 1960s, based on a Beveridgian model of universal, public, tax-funded coverage of hospital and physician services. Under the Canadian constitution, health care is the responsibility of the provinces and territories. However, in 1966, the federal government set out five principles for implementing a national health care system: public administration, comprehensiveness, universality, portability (between provinces), and accessibility (introduced later in 1984). Although not responsible for the delivery of health care, the federal government used its spending power to introduce the public health care system and committed to partially fund provinces that complied with those principles. Hospital services are delivered through public or not-for-profit organizations. Physicians work mostly in private clinics and are paid directly by the government without overbilling.

The province of Québec set up its system in 1971 with the full integration of health and social services at the local, regional, and provincial levels. Locally, services are provided via hospitals, rehabilitation centers, youth centers, and nursing homes. In addition, Local Community Services Centers (Centres locaux de services

[1] This text is a short version of a book chapter previously published: Hébert R. Canada: Application of a Coordinated-Type Integration Model for Vulnerable Older People in Québec: The PRISMA Project. In Amelung V, Stein V, Goodwin N, Balicer R, Nolte E & Suter (eds), Springer: Cham (Switzerland), 2017.

communautaires (CLSC)) were designed to be the primary care portal for health and social services in the community. Private for-profit operations are virtually non-existent in the Québec health care system, except for residential facilities for older people. Voluntary agencies are well developed, particularly for home services. Social economy agencies (not for profit) are also very active in providing support for domestic tasks and personal care.

The population of Canada and Québec is aging quickly. In 2014, 17% of the population (1.4 million people) in Québec was over 65 years old. Since the baby boom in the 1950s, particularly in the French-speaking Québec population, it has been expected that older people will make up over 25% of the population by 2031. Despite the integration of health and social services, delivering services to a growing vulnerable older population was a challenge. Prior to 2003, many public organizations (hospitals, nursing homes, rehabilitation centers, CLSCs), together with social economy and voluntary agencies, delivered care without coordination. Multiple assessments, delays, redundant services, gaps in services, and multiple providers created inefficiencies, compromised service quality, and increased costs, probably unduly. There was a pressing need to integrate those services.

PRISMA (Program of Research to Integrate Services for the Maintenance of Autonomy)[2] is a coordinated-type integration model developed by a steering committee, including policymakers at the provincial and regional levels, health care managers, clinicians, and researchers. The coordination level of integration was originally suggested by Leutz [3] as one of three types of integration (in addition to liaison and full integration), but at that time, there was no model developed to operationalize it. Unlike fully integrated systems, this model includes all public, private, and voluntary health and social service organizations involved in caring for older people in a given area. Each organization keeps its own structure but agrees to participate under an umbrella system and to adapt its operations and resources to agreed requirements and processes. At this level, the integrated service delivery system is not just nested in the health care and social services system (like fully integrated models); it is embedded within it.

The PRISMA model comprises six components: (1) coordination between decision-makers and managers at the regional and local levels, (2) a single entry point with a case-finding tool (Prisma-7 [9]), (3) case management, (4) individualized service plans [10], (5) a single assessment instrument (the SMAF) [11] coupled with a case-mix management system (the Iso-SMAF Profiles) [12, 13] computerized clinical chart [13]. Figure 1.1 summarizes the model.

After being pretested with promising results [14], the PRISMA model was implemented in July 2001 in three regions of the Eastern Townships in the province of Québec (one urban and two rural). The PRISMA model was subject to rigorous

[2]All the publications on the PRISMA model and experiments, in both French and English are available on the following website: http://www.prisma-qc.ca/cgi-cs/cs.waframe.index?lang=2.

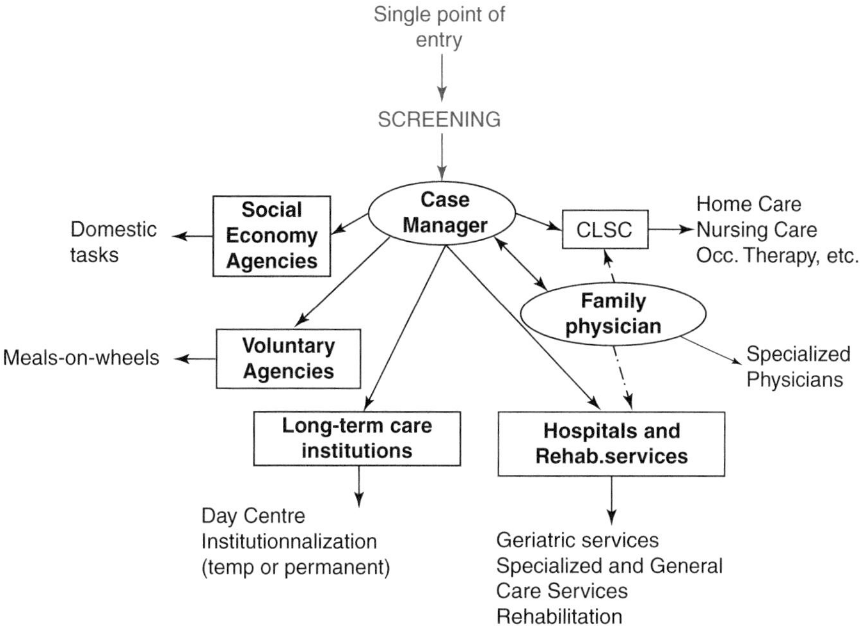

Fig. 1.1 Flow of patients through the coordinated PRISMA model (reproduced with permission from the Journal of Integrated Care—Emerald Group)

evaluation, including an implementation study that sought to monitor the degree and process of implementation, and an outcome study, using a longitudinal (4 years) population-based quasi-experimental design with three experimental and three comparison areas.

Over the last 2 years of experimental implementation (when the implementation rate was over 70% [15], there was a 6% reduction of functional decline (62 fewer cases per 1000 individuals) in the experimental groups ($p < 0.05$). In the fourth year of the study, the annual incidence of functional decline dropped by 14% in the experimental groups (137 cases per 1000; $p < 0.001$), while the prevalence of unmet needs in the comparison regions was nearly double the prevalence observed in the experimental regions ($p < 0.001$). Satisfaction and empowerment were significantly higher in the experimental groups ($p < 0.001$). For health service utilization, fewer visits to emergency rooms ($p < 0.001$) and hospitalizations ($p = 0.11$) than expected were observed in the experimental cohorts [16]. An economic analysis comparing the cost of care in the experimental groups, including the cost of the PRISMA component, to the comparison groups showed that the costs were similar. This means that the PRISMA model was more efficient than the usual care.

During the study in 2003, the Québec Minister of Health was convinced that the model would be successful (even before the results were formally published) and decided to undertake a major health care reform merging the different public organizations involved in caring for older people within a local area (hospitals, nursing homes, and home care organizations) in the CSSSs (Health and Social Services Centers) [17]. This structural integration was seen by the Minister as providing strong support for improving the coordination of services. However, as demonstrated in other contexts, structural integration does not necessarily foster functional integration [18]. The reverse was actually observed in Québec over the first 4 years of the reform. The implementation rate of the PRISMA model, based on the same indicators developed in the experiment, was only on average 38% in 2008, although a wider rollout of the PRISMA model was included in the Ministry's 2005–2010 action plan [19]. The rollout of the PRISMA model was slowed considerably and was even stopped momentarily in many regions because, first, the CSSSs' different programs continued to work in silos and, second, this new big organization in the system (the CSSS) no longer prioritized coordination committees and collaboration with voluntary agencies, social economy enterprises, and private providers that are also involved in delivering services to frail older people [20]. Nevertheless, after 10 years, the implementation of the PRISMA model reached 70% across the province in 2014 (Fig. 1.2).

In 2015, a new structural reform was implemented in Québec, merging all the public institutions in a region, including rehabilitation and youth centers. These new *Integrated* Health and Social Services Centers (CISSSs) replaced also the regional authorities. Although improving integrated services was one of the reasons for the reform, this new structural integration has negative impacts on functional integration, as was the case in the 2003 reform.

The PRISMA model has been adopted in other countries (France [21, 22] and Spain) and populations (young patients with mental and physical disabilities). In

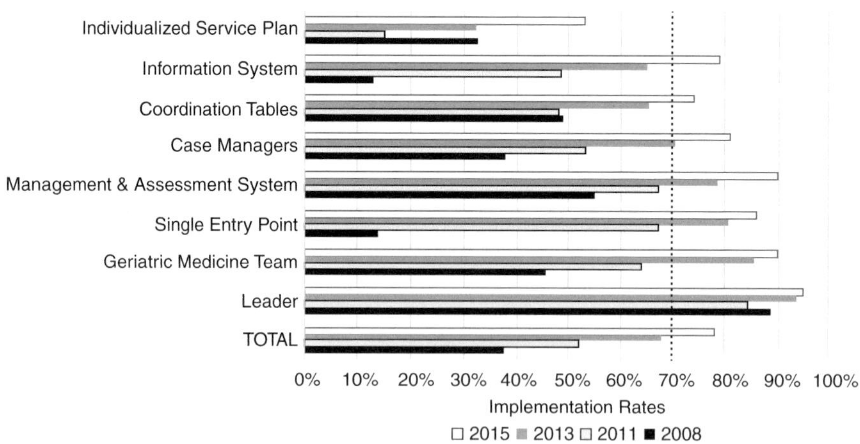

Fig. 1.2 Implementation rates of the PRISMA model in Québec, Canada, from 2008 to 2015

PRISMA, a necessary seventh component was not included in the model, namely financing, which is usually one component of integrated models [23]. The implementation of a long-term care insurance scheme would support the operationalization of the PRISMA model [24, 25].

Germany

Germany's Older Population

At the end of 2019, the population of Germany reached a new high of 83.2 million people. One person in four is at least 60 years old, while one person in five is at least 67 years old and thus of pensionable age [26]. The older group spans several age decades; it is extraordinarily heterogeneous and is going to continue to grow. This demographic change is happening in urban and rural regions in equal measure and has been apparent for a long time [27]. More and more older adults are considerably healthier, more satisfied, and more vital in their current living situation than previous generations have been [28]. They feel, on average, up to 10 years younger than the calendar says they are [29]. Living in one's own home (the traditional way of living) is one of the central concerns in old age and provides an important indicator of independence. About 95% of older adults in Germany live alone or with their spouse or partner in a private household [26]. Innovative ways of living, such as multigenerational households and communities for older people in need of care or people with dementia, are still the exception [30]. The best-known new way of living, now found throughout Germany, is the relatively independent serviced living model in accommodation complexes, which are architecturally barrier-free and have communal rooms and activities [31].

The Seventh Government Report on the Situation of Older People: Care and Shared Responsibility in the Municipal Community

The report found that the development of local structures and designing an environment meeting the needs of older people rests primarily with the local authorities. One of the principles in this process is the principle of subsidiarity, emphasizing the involvement of local structures and networks. The second is the German Social Code (SGB), which is based on the federal system, to achieve "social justice and security." [32] The third is the local authorities' responsibility for *Daseinsvorsorge*. This concept does refer to public services for daily life, also called "essential public services" or "services of general interest."

Health Promotion and Provision and Care for Older People in the Context of Community-Based Integrated Care

The Social Code (SGB) regulates such areas as insurance against unemployment and occupational incapacity, pension insurance, health insurance, and care insurance.

The health funds (*Krankenkassen*) have the task of maintaining, restoring, and improving the health state of insured people, including the promotion of health competence. This was strengthened by a legal amendment on primary disease prevention and health promotion (PrävG) [33].

Treatment by general practitioners (GPs) and specialists, including vaccinations and preventive checkups (e.g., Check-up 35+ and cancer prevention) are provided locally, close to people's homes. Acute geriatric hospital treatment provided on an in-patient or outpatient basis and geriatric rehabilitation meets the different levels of need for local geriatric care. Some geriatric hospitals provide ambulatory or mobile geriatric rehabilitation. In addition, there are outpatient clinics in hospital geriatric departments. The results of comprehensive geriatric assessments are used for individual treatment plans, which are provided to the doctor (GP or any other physician) who referred the patient to the service.

The "Integrated provision" concept provides another way of overcoming the borders between the community-based and hospital-based sectors, though only in specific situations and for limited periods of time. Statutory health funds may offer individual contracts with different health care and social care providers, medical device manufacturers, etc. in order to offer "Integrated provision," which includes preventive or curative rehabilitation in addition to legally defined standard services.

Another part of the Social Code regulates social care insurance for everyone who is insured with statutory health funds. This insurance provides assistance to people who are dependent on support because of the severity of their condition. Subsidiarity is a basic principle, and the initial responsibility rests with the family. The need for care is assessed in a standardized way in the applicant's home by the statutory health funds' medical service (MDK). About 10% of people aged 60 years or older are assessed to need some level of care. The need for care does not arise greatly until very old age; around two-thirds of people over 90 years old are in need of care. The vast majority of older people live in their own homes with support from visiting carers [34].

Prospects for Building Community-Based Integrated Care for Older People

Older people's independence and quality of life are decided primarily by their biological age and their functional competence. Frailty and loss of function (disability) limit their potential for self-help and also limit their options with regard to independent living and social participation [35]. The central question is how to recognize developing losses of function as early as possible so that appropriate measures can be put in place to maintain independence. Findings from the Longitudinal Urban Cohort Ageing Study (LUCAS) show the importance of functional resources and risks in old age and point to opportunities for taking early action to promote health and prevent illness before help and care become necessary [36]. Simple filtering processes (screenings) using short self-completed questionnaires, such as the LUCAS functional ability index, and also performance testing with tasks relevant to daily life make it possible to identify older people with risk factors. This can be done in such settings as sports clubs, community meeting rooms, senior citizens' clubs, pharmacies, and GP practices. Any risks or problems identified should be seen as a reason to take appropriate measures. Examples can be found in the LUCAS NAVIGATOR: https://www.albertinen.de/fileadmin/Media/Medizin_Gesundheit/AH/Geriatrische_Forschungsabteilung/LUCAS/Lucas_Navigator_2020_englisch.pdf.

It is imperative to develop functional competence in order to maintain health, particularly among the large group of independent and active older people living in the community (those classed as robust/postrobust by the LUCAS functional ability index). The "Active health promotion in old age" program aimed to achieve this. It was carried out in small groups at a geriatric center by an interdisciplinary team of health advice experts and focused on medical screening, nutrition, movement, and social participation [37]. For 13.8 years, this long-term program had significant positive effects, compressing morbidity and improving survival [38].

The model project "Living independently in your neighborhood for longer" (NWGA) is supported by the G-BA "Innovation fund." The project has set up a coordination point in a geriatric center to provide case management. Older people with limitations of function (prefrail/frail on the LUCAS functional ability index) or losses of function (requiring care according to MDK) receive a comprehensive geriatric assessment and an individual support plan. Participants are also offered the use of a tablet computer as a technical assistance system. The results of the acceptance analysis will be interesting; up to now, those who are frail and in need of care—for whom ambient assisted living (AAL) programs are intended to improve the quality of life at home—have tended to feel that such technical assistance systems are not for them [39].

The Hamburg home visiting program has chosen a different path. On reaching their 80th birthday, all citizens of the state of Hamburg (about 17,000 people each year) receive a free individual home visit to inform them about the local health and support services available. If they are interested in any of the services (e.g., home alterations, local advice for older people, care support), the necessary arrangements are made.

Multisector local networks and cooperation structures are needed to nurture these efforts in the long term. The Hamburg State Health and Consumer Protection Authority is involved in the European innovation partnership platform EIP AHA "Active and Healthy Ageing" (https://ec.europa.eu/eip/ageing/home_en) with best practice examples in "Falls prevention" (A2) and "Age friendly environments"

(D4). In 2018, the "Age friendly environments" action group, actors, and stakeholders involved throughout Europe came together in Hamburg. One of the topics under discussion was MINDMAP, a research project being carried out by a European consortium on "Promoting mental well-being and healthy aging in cities." MINDMAP has collected data on the conditions surrounding health promotion, disease prevention, and care and also on networking activities in 12 European cities. This survey reveals the great variety of community-based integrated care activities in Hamburg and the other MINDMAP cities with established long-term urban cohort aging studies [40].

The Hamburg State Health and Consumer Protection Authority also coordinate "Prevention pact—working together to keep Hamburg healthy." In 2010, the authority established a cooperative alliance with over 120 partner institutions; the alliance aims to achieve "Healthy aging in Hamburg" and to reinforce health promotion and the prevention of illness among older people in different settings (https://www.hamburg.de/pakt-fuer-praevention/). These examples demonstrate the central role played by municipal communities in transforming health and care provision in innovative ways to establish reliable community-based integrated care for older people.

Japan

Japan is experiencing unprecedented aging of its population. People aged 65 years or older accounted for 28.4% of the total population in 2019, and that proportion is expected to reach a plateau in 2040–2050 (approximately 40%). In 2018, the average life expectancy was 81.25 years for men and 87.32 years for women. Additionally, people aged 85 years or older are approximately 6 million and will reach 10 million in 2040, when the total population in Japan will be approximately 100 million. Thus, we will live in a society where approximately 1 out of 10 will be 85 years or older. The number of disabled older adults (care level 1 to 5 based on the long-term care insurance system) and those living alone is 4.71 million in 2019 and 5.93 million in 2015, respectively, and the number will increase dramatically.

As the country's demographics change, the disease structure changes, and therefore the demand for medical care changes. The Japanese government launched the long-term care insurance system in 2000 [41, 42], responding to the rapidly aging population with its rising care needs. This policy provides a variety of home, community-based, and institutional services to which every older Japanese person is entitled based on their physical and mental status.

In addition, future demands for medical care will accelerate the transition to health care and nursing care services for dementia, frailty, sarcopenia, and other geriatric syndromes [43]. In addition to acute medical care, the provision of health care and nursing care needs to be considered for the convalescent and chronic stages of conditions, which are provided in convalescent rehabilitation facilities and several types of nursing homes and home care. In this environment, it is not sufficient for us to provide medical care for older people that merely deals with each disease in a fragmented manner. A broad perspective that considers the function of all organs, activities of daily living (ADL), frailty, and environmental factors is required. With these in mind, the Japanese government proposed the establishment of a "Community-based Integrated Care System" by 2025, when baby boomers will become age 75 or older [44]. The purpose of this system is to comprehensively ensure the provision of health care, nursing care, preventive care, housing, and livelihood support in each community. Home medical care is also the cornerstone of health care in a community-based integrated care system, and the promotion of this field is undoubtedly important in promoting community-based integrated care. It is also important to note that various home-based services, such as home-visit nursing and nursing care, play a very important role in community-based integrated care, along with home medical care. On the other hand, home medical care is still developing and needs to be further developed, considering future demand. Constructing a comprehensive home medical care system in Japan is a huge challenge and an indispensable milestone for aging in place.

In 2006, the government implemented measures aimed to identify frail or prefrail older adults and provide early preventive care programs for the prevention of functional decline and to delay dependence on long-term care. The measures consisted of identifying older people with disability risks by screening them using a validated questionnaire (Kihon Checklist) [45]. The identified frail or prefrail older persons were subsequently referred to community prevention programs for free. However, the utilization of the Kihon Checklist was not enough to identify high-risk individuals for disability, and participation in the local intervention programs was quite low. Based on screening by the Kihon Checklist, the government estimated that approximately 5% of the older population who received screening was at risk and should be the target of preventive care. However, in 2014, by the ninth year of strategy implementation, only 0.8% of older adults had joined the community prevention program, which was unexpectedly low [46]. This result was due to the low participation in the screening process for functional difficulties: only 34.8% of older people participated [47]. We speculate that physical and environmental barriers and the lack of support to overcome these barriers, such as incentives and transportation, may explain the low participation. In addition, low awareness of disability prevention among general practitioners as well as the general public might have affected the outcome. The low participation in the community prevention programs resulted in limited attributable impact. However, we have shown the effect of the prevention program if the program is appropriately managed [48]. The government recognized difficulties in maintaining participants' motivation and hence changed its policies for population-based preventive service provision.

With extensive efforts for disability prevention after the implementation of the long-term care insurance system, public long-term care prevention plans now focus on promoting social participation and preventing the isolation of older people, since isolation has been identified as a strong risk factor for disability and mortality [49]. In 2015, the government reformed the Long-Term Care Insurance Act by changing its primary strategy for long-term care prevention from a high-risk strategy to a community-based population strategy, targeting the general population regardless of the risk level. The new strategy aims to build a community that can seamlessly provide preventive, medical, and long-term care, welfare, and housing services to all individuals. Based on the population strategy for long-term care prevention, central and local governments have promoted community activities, such as salons, to facilitate group participation and encourage social activities among older adults.

Shifting from a high-risk strategy to a population strategy involving multidisciplinary community collaborations has been successful in Japan in the sense that a larger number of older people participated in the preventive program. For community-based integrated care systems to succeed, a collaboration between community members and diverse service providers is mandatory. Collaboration allows community members to create or modify their own community welfare services in line with their needs and local situations. Quantitative health equity assessments and visualizing the results in an easily understandable manner are also useful in identifying and prioritizing problems, as well as sharing community goals of local actions and policies with service providers and community members. In 2017, the World Health Organization (WHO) published the Guidelines on Integrated Care for Older People (ICOPE) to provide guidance on preventing, slowing, or reversing the decline of the intrinsic capabilities of older individuals and maximizing their functional abilities [50]. The guidelines make evidence-based recommendations for the comprehensive assessment of the health status of older people and the delivery of integrated health care. Most of the guideline recommendations involve secondary prevention measures, that is, identifying frail older people and providing them with preventive care. However, as supported by Japan's experience, secondary prevention measures or the screening of frail individuals needs effective screening measures to identify frail individuals, effective interventions to mitigate possible risks, and effective means to deliver the intervention to frail individuals. Integrated care for long-term care prevention should include more community-based interventions for the whole community. To build local organizational networks for providing such care, health care professionals and organizations should be actively involved.

South Korea

South Korea has a rapidly aging population, where the percentage of those aged 65 years or older is projected to increase from 14.9% in 2019 to 43.9% by 2060 [51]. The older population is also aging, with the 75+ age group's share increasing from 43.5% to 62.9% in the same period. With the rapid population aging, older Koreans' demand for an array of services covering health, long-term, and social care is increasing. Older Koreans overwhelmingly prefer to age in place, with 88.6% preferring to stay in their homes when in good health and 57.6% still favoring their current residence when functionally impaired. However, many are institutionalized as they become frail in part because of insufficient and underdeveloped community resources. Stimulated by the substantially rising costs of care in acute and long-term institutions, the proportion of total health care expenditures consumed by the older population is projected to increase from 38.7% in 2016 to 50.8% by 2025. Finding ways to expand community-based services delivered in an integrated manner has become critical in helping older people live in their community as well as in reducing the costs of inappropriate institutionalizations.

Historically, the development of community-based integrated care in Korea has been approached from two perspectives on service integration. One focuses on *the integration of health care and long-term care*, where the establishment of a publicly-funded health and long-term care insurance system has primarily driven the discussion. The other has centered on *the integration of health care and social care*, where local governments have introduced various models of integrated care in the community. Over the years, the two paths for establishing community-based integrated care have been slowly merging. They have recently taken form as a major policy initiative in which both the central and municipal governments are paving the way for coordinated delivery of health care, long-term care, and social care in the community.

The financing structure plays a crucial role in determining the coordination between service providers. The National Health Insurance, achieving universal coverage since 1989, and the National Long-term Care Insurance, introduced in 2008, have been the largest sources of public financing for health care and long-term care, respectively [52]. Although the two public insurance systems are funded separately, the National Health Insurance Service (NHIS) administers both insurance schemes to reduce administrative costs. Recently, there have been calls for better integration between health care and long-term care services for older people because of the lack of coordination between the two service sectors, the inadequate provision of health services for older residents in the community and long-term care facilities, and the overlapping and inefficient use of resources by health and long-term care institutions [53]. Because of the separate funding mechanism for health care and long-term care, pooling funds and organizing services pose a significant challenge, made worse by the absence of care managers. Home health care, such as home-visit nursing services, are not readily available and are underutilized. The overlapping function of long-term care hospitals and facilities results in inefficiency. Older people who are frail but not eligible for long-term care insurance are referred to the community for support, registered to receive a range of health and social care, including preventive health services, home-visit nursing, adult day care, in-home supportive services, and meal delivery [54]. However, many regions lack capacity or resources, resulting in services that are often inadequate or inaccessible.

Efforts to integrate health and social care in the community have concentrated mainly on public initiatives from local governments and agencies. Since 1995, the municipal government has experimented with different models for delivering integrated care for community-dwelling older adults. At the district level, nurses were teamed up with social workers in the Health and Welfare Office set up within the community health care centers to provide home visiting services jointly. This approach to the structural integration of health and social care, which lasted for 4 years, although attaining increased understanding and sharing of information between the two disparate professionals, did not result in active linkages or coordination of health care and social services [55].

The less than satisfactory results of the strategy to consolidate health and social organizations led to a toned-down approach [56]. Between 2000 and 2003, a linkage-type model was designed and implemented in two major cities in Gyeonggi Province surrounding the capital, Seoul. The Health and Welfare Linkage Center for Older People was set up in the provincial medical center, composed of a team of physicians, nurses, social workers, and administrative personnel. The multidisciplinary team was involved not in providing direct services but in identifying older adults' needs and orchestrating health and social resources in the community through information sharing between providers. The center's role as a liaison between services increased service linkages and helped reduce overlapping and unnecessary services. However, unmet needs remained, especially for health care, including referral to hospitals, home-visit nursing, emergency medical service, rehabilitation, and mental health [57].

As part of the effort to plan and implement integrated community care across districts and towns, the Community Security Council was established in 2005 [58]. This local governance structure serves to plan and organize not only services related to social and health care but also resources on employment, housing, education, culture, and environment from both public and private sectors to deliver to community residents. Public-private partnerships are fostered to form cooperative networks across diverse provider groups, including local welfare centers, public health centers, and general physician's offices. Emphasis is placed on hiring social workers and nurses to expand case management and home visiting services, especially for at-risk community residents.

More recently, two notable public initiatives were set in motion. One is the 301 Network, located in a public medical center in the northern part of Seoul, which links medical care and social care services [59]. The integrated health and social care support center, consisting of a team of physicians, nurses, and social workers, functions to identify and assess the vulnerable population and provide linkages to community resources. A diverse set of services are provided, including home visits by a team of physicians, nurses, and social workers; formal caregiver support; referral to hospitals; care management (health checkups, polypharmacy, linkages to community services); and meal delivery. The 365 Network, an offshoot of the 301 Network, focuses on people aged 60 years or older, providing posthospital discharge monitoring and management, special meals (type 2 diabetes meal plan and low-salt diet), and home environment modifications to ensure safety.

Since 2015, the Seoul metropolitan government has been transforming town offices into "outreach community centers." These centers were reinforced with social workers and home-visiting nurses working as a team to enable the care management of community residents, especially those who fall through the cracks in the public safety net, including older people. Linkage to health and social services has increased throughout the years with high levels of satisfaction among the residents. However, maintaining qualified nursing personnel and mobilizing private community resources has proven difficult [60].

Efforts to integrate health care and long-term care, brought on by the establishment of the social insurance system and the development of community models to integrate health care and social care and which sprouted at the municipal level, culminated in a joint initiative by the central and local governments, the Community Integrated Care Demonstration Project, introduced in 2018. Initially starting as a demonstration project in eight counties and expanding to 16 since, it addresses four key areas: (1) housing (building care-friendly public rental apartments, supporting home improvement for independent living and fall prevention, and promoting urban redevelopment conducive to community care), (2) health care (providing home-based primary care, community-based chronic disease management, community health promotion and preventive services, and hospital discharge planning), (3) long-term care (expanding home- and community-based services and providing postdischarge community living support for the low-income group), and (4) service linkages (promoting better integration between health and welfare information systems, supporting the development of integrated care models based on public-private partnerships, expanding the care management workforce). Restructuring the current service delivery system to attain better coordination of different types of services, enhancing cooperation between primary care physicians and home care nurses, and pooling health care and long-term care insurance with local government funds are among the issues that need to be resolved [61].

Summary

In response to the currently fragmented care system that fails to meet the diverse needs of older community residents, models of community-based integrated care are being developed. In this chapter, we examined cases from four countries across North America, Europe, and East Asia. Each country brings a unique perspective to developing community-based health and long-term care services for older adults. Unlike the full-integration model of the Program of All-Inclusive Care for the Elderly (PACE) in the United States, a coordination-type model has been implemented and intensively evaluated in Canada. In Germany, the responsibility of designing community-based integrated care rests primarily on the local authorities, with the organization of various health and long-term care services grounded in the nation's policy toward solidarity and its strong public insurance system. Japan has launched a comprehensive care system to provide home medical care, nursing care, housing, and living support to older people in the community. South Korea, as a newcomer to the field, has recently laid out an ambitious plan to build up community care systems in towns across the country.

Some commonalities emerge in the approach to integrating care in the community. These include coordination between and within various stakeholders, including policymakers and providers; care planning and management through an interdisciplinary team; a public financing system; and the delegation of responsibilities to localities or regions for the organization and delivery of services. Establishing community-based integrated care is a long-term process beset by challenges, as many models developed over the years have failed to scale up. Insufficient funding, inappropriate allocation of resources, limited long-range capacity building and planning, and the rigid nature of the current care system for coordinating a broad range of services have constituted major obstacles in developing integrated models of community-based care. One of the lessons learned from implementing innovative models is that structural integration does not automatically lead to functional integration, as is evident in the case of Canada and Korea. Recent attempts in Japan and Korea, where establishing "care-friendly" communities that incorporate housing and living support as critical components, are closely being watched. A public health approach taken in Germany and Japan, with an emphasis on healthy aging through the dissemination of health promotion and prevention programs in the community, may well prove to be a feasible strategy to reduce the demand for services in the long run.

It is difficult to predict whether recent innovations in coordinating care across a broad spectrum of different services will have a lasting impact and be financially sustainable. As countries expand community-based integrated care, we will see whether care can indeed come "home."

References

1. Plochg T, Klazinga NS. Community-based integrated care: myth or must? Int J Qual Health Care. 2002;14(2):91–101.
2. Valentijn PP, Schepman SM, Opheij W, Bruijnzeels MA. Understanding integrated care: a comprehensive conceptual framework based on the integrative functions of primary care. Int J Integr Care. 2013;13:e010.
3. Leutz WN. Five laws for integrating medical and social services: lessons from the United States and the United Kingdom. Milbank Q. 1999;77(1):77–110.
4. Goodwin N, Stein V, Amelung V. Chapter 1. What is integrated care? In: Amelung V, Stein V, Goodwin N, Balicer R, Nolte E, Suter E, editors. Handbook integrated care. Cham: Springer; 2017. https://doi.org/10.1007/978-3-319-56103-5_1.
5. Baxter S, Johnson M, Chambers D, Sutton A, Goyder E, Booth A. The effects of integrated care: a systematic review of UK and international evidence. BMC Health Serv Res. 2018;18:350.
6. Leichsenring K, Alaszewski AM, editors. Providing integrated health and social care for older persons. Burlington: Ashgate; 2004.
7. WHO Regional Office for Europe. Integrated care models: an overview. Copenhagen: WHO Regional Office for Europe; 2016.
8. Béland F, Hollander MJ. Integrated models of care delivery for the frail elderly: international perspectives. Gac Sanit. 2011;25(Suppl 2):138–46.
9. Raîche M, Hébert R, Dubois MF. PRISMA-7: a case-finding tool to identify older adults with moderate to severe disabilities. Arch Gerontol Geriatr. 2008;47(1):9–18.
10. Somme D, Bonin L, Lebel P, Hébert R, Blanchard F. Development of an individualized service plan tool and rules for case management in Québec. Care Manag J. 2009;10(3):89–99.
11. Hébert R, Carrier R, Bilodeau A. The functional autonomy measurement system (SMAF): description and validation of an instrument for the measurement of handicaps. Age Ageing. 1988;17:293–302.

12. Dubuc N, Hébert R, Desrosiers J, Buteau M, Trottier L. Disability-based classification system for older people in integrated long-term care services: the Iso-SMAF profiles. Arch Gerontol Geriatr. 2006;42:191–206.
13. Hébert R, Dubois MF, Dubuc N, Tousignant M, Raîche M, Veil A. Evaluation of the implementation of PRISMA, a coordination-type integrated service delivery system for frail older people in Quebec. J Integr Care. 2008;16(6):4–14.
14. Tourigny A, Durand P, Bonin L, Hébert R, Rochette L. Quasi-experimental study of the effectiveness of an integrated service delivery network for the frail elderly. Can J Aging. 2004;23:231–46.
15. Hébert R, Veil A. Monitoring the degree of implementation of an integrated delivery system. Int J Integr Care. 2004;4:1–11.
16. Hébert R, Raîche M, Dubois MF, Gueye NR, Dubuc N, Tousignant M. Impact of PRISMA, a coordination-type integrated service delivery system for frail older people in Quebec (Canada): a quasi-experimental study. J Gerontol Ser B Soc Sci. 2010;65:107–18.
17. Levine D. The reform of health and social services in Quebec. Healthc Pap. 2007;8:46–54.
18. Demers L. Mergers and integrated care: the Quebec experience. Int J Integr Care. 2013;13:e002.
19. Gouvernement du Québec. Un défi de solidarité: Les services aux aînés en perte d'autonomie. Plan d'action 2005-2010. Québec; 2005.
20. INSPQ. Synthèse des connaissances sur les conditions de mise en œuvre des réseaux de services intégrés aux personnes âgées. Québec: Institut national de santé publique du Québec; 2014.
21. République française. Quality labelling throughout the country for "single points of contact", the "Maisons pour l'Autonomie et l'Intégration des malades Alzheimer" (MAIA); 2008. http://www.plan-alzheimer.gouv.fr/measure-no4.html.
22. Somme D, Trouvé H, Couturier Y, Carrier S, Gagnon D, Lavallart B, Hébert R, Cretin C, Saint-Jean O. Prisma France: implementation program of an innovation in health and services system for disabled people. Adaptation of a case-management based integration model. Rev Epidemiol Sante Publique. 2008;56:54–62.
23. Kodner DL. Whole-system approaches to health and social care partnerships for the frail elderly: an exploration of North American models and lessons. Health Soc Care Community. 2006;14:384–90.
24. Hébert R. Public long-term care insurance: a way to ensure sustainable continuity of care for frail older people. Healthc Pap. 2011;11(1):69–75.
25. Hébert R. Still-born autonomy insurance plan in Quebec: example of a public long-term care insurance system in Canada. Healthc Pap. 2016;15(4):45–50. https://doi.org/10.12927/hcpap.2016.24589.
26. Statistisches Bundesamt. Bevölkerung im Wandel. Annahmen und Ergebnisse der 14. koordinierten Bevölkerungsvorausberechnung. Wiesbaden; 2019. https://www.destatis.de/DE/Publikationen/Thematisch/Bevoelkerung/VorausberechnungBevoelkerung/BevoelkerungDeutschland2060Presse5124204159004.pdf?__blob=publicationFile. Accessed on May 1, 2020.
27. Bundesministerium für Familie, Senioren, Frauen und Jugend (BMFSFJ). Vierter Altenbericht zur Lage der älteren Generation in der Bundesrepublik Deutschland – Risiken, Lebensqualität und Versorgung Hochaltriger –unter besonderer Berücksichtigung demenzieller Erkrankungen und Stellungnahme der Bundesregierung. Berlin; 2002. https://www.bmfsfj.de/bmfsfj/service/publikationen/4-altenbericht-/95594. Accessed on May 1, 2020.
28. Bundesministerium für Familie, Senioren, Frauen und Jugend (BMFSFJ). A new culture of ageing: images of ageing in society. Findings and recommendations of the Sixth German Government Report on the Elderly. Berlin; 2010. https://www.bmfsfj.de/blob/93188/729a35d76df46edf3aba263085b2e121/6-altenbericht-eine-neue-kultur des alterns englisch-data.pdf. Accessed on May 1, 2020.
29. Generali Zukunftsfonds und Institut für Demoskopie Allensbach. Generali-Altersstudie. Wie ältere Menschen leben, denken und sich engagieren. Frankfurt am Main: Fischer Taschenbuch Verlag; 2013.

30. Wahl HW, Steiner B. Innovative Wohnformen. In: Pantel J, Schröder J, Bollheimer C, Sieber C, Kruse A, editors. Praxishandbuch Altersmedizin. Geriatrie – Gerontopsychiatrie - Gerontologie. Stuttgart: Kohlhammer Verlag; 2014. p. 701–7.
31. Jacobs K, Kuhlmey A, Greß S, Einführung SA. Pflege-report 2015. Schwerpunkt: Pflege zwischen Heim und Häuslichkeit. Stuttgart: Schattauer-Verlag; 2015. p. XII–XVII.
32. Bundesministerium für Familie, Senioren, Frauen und Jugend (BMFSFJ). Care and shared responsibility in the municipal community. Findings and recommendations of the seventh report on the elderly. Berlin; 2016. https://www.bmfsfj.de/bmfsfj/meta/en/publications-en/care-and-shared-responsibility-in-the-municipal-community/120958. Accessed on May 1, 2020.
33. Nationale Präventionskonferenz. Bundesrahmenempfehlungen der Nationalen Präventionskonferenz nach § 20d Abs. 3 SGB V, extended version. Berlin; 2018. https://www.npk-info.de/fileadmin/user_upload/ueber_die_npk/downloads/1_bundesrahmenempfehlung/bundesrahmenempfehlung_BRE_praevention_barrierefrei.pdf.
34. Statistisches Bundesamt. Pflegestatistik 2017. Pflege im Rahmen der Pflegeversicherung – Deutschlandergebnisse. Wiesbaden; 2018. https://www.destatis.de/DE/Themen/Gesellschaft-Umwelt/Gesundheit/Pflege/_inhalt.html. Accessed May 1, 2020.
35. World Health Organization. World Health Report on ageing and health. Luxembourg; 2015. http://apps.who.int/iris/bitstream/10665/186463/1/9789240694811_eng.pdf?ua=1. Accessed May 1, 2020.
36. Dapp U, Minder C, Anders J, Golgert S, von Renteln-Kruse W. Long-term prediction of changes in health status, frailty, nursing care and mortality in community-dwelling senior citizens - results from the Longitudinal Urban Cohort Ageing Study (LUCAS). BMC Geriatr. 2014;14:141.
37. Dapp U, Anders J, von Renteln-Kruse W, Meier-Baumgartner HP. Active health promotion in old age: methodology of a preventive intervention programme provided by an interdisciplinary health advisory team for independent older people. J Public Health. 2005;13:122–7.
38. Dapp U, Minder CE, Neumann L, Golgert S, Klugmann B, von Renteln-Kruse W. Effectiveness of "Active health promotion in old age": results regarding compression of morbidity by target groups in 13.8 years of observation in LUCAS. Z Gerontol Geriatr. 2018;51:379–87.
39. Dapp U, Anders J. Open-minded? Older people's attitude regarding ambient assisted living. Preference analysis based on 1,430 participants of the Longitudinal Urban Cohort Ageing Study (LUCAS). Psychother Alter. 2020;17:25–48.
40. Neumann L, Dapp U, Jacobsen W, van Lenthe F, von Renteln-Kruse W. The MINDMAP project: mental well-being in urban environments. Design and first results of a survey on healthcare planning policies, strategies and programmes that address mental health promotion and mental disorder prevention for older people in Europe. Z Gerontol Geriatr. 2017;50:588–602.
41. Tsutsui T, Muramatsu N. Care-needs certification in the long-term care insurance system of Japan. J Am Geriatr Soc. 2005 Mar;53(3):522–7.
42. Morikawa M. Towards community-based integrated care: trends and issues in Japan's long-term care policy. Int J Integr Care. 2014;14:e005.
43. Arai H, Ouchi Y, Toba K, Endo T, Shimokado K, Tsubota K, et al. Japan as the front-runner of super-aged societies: perspectives from medicine and medical care in Japan. Geriatr Gerontol Int. 2015;15(6):673–87.
44. Tsutsui T. Implementation process and challenges for the community-based integrated care system in Japan. Int J Integr Care. 2014;14:e002.
45. Tsuji T, Kondo K, Kondo N, Aida J, Takagi D. Development of a risk assessment scale predicting incident functional disability among older people: Japan Gerontological Evaluation Study. Geriatr Gerontol Int. 2018;18(10):1433–8.
46. The survey for implementation of long-term care prevention programmes and preventive everyday living support comprehensive programmes. Tokyo: Ministry of Health, Labour, and Welfare; 2014. https://www.mhlw.go.jp/file/06-Seisakujouhou-12300000-Roukenkyoku/0000077238_3.pdf.

47. Saito J, Haseda M, Amemiya A, Takagi D, Kondo K, Kondo N. Community-based care for healthy ageing: lessons from Japan. Bull World Health Organ. 2019;97(8):570–4.
48. Yamada M, Arai H, Sonoda T, Aoyama T. Community-based exercise program is cost-effective by preventing care and disability in Japanese frail older adults. J Am Med Dir Assoc. 2012;13(6):507–11.
49. Saito M, Kondo N, Kondo K, Ojima T, Hirai H. Gender differences on the impacts of social exclusion on mortality among older Japanese: AGES cohort study. Soc Sci Med. 2012;75(5):940–5.
50. Guidelines on integrated care for older people. Geneva: World Health Organization (ICOPE); 2017. https://www.who.int/ageing/publications/guidelines-icope/en/.
51. Kim JS, Nam KC, Park SK, Shin DI. Strategies for implementing community care policy. Seoul: The Presidential Committee on Policy and Strategy; 2019.
52. National Health Insurance Service. National health insurance system of Korea. Wonju: National Health Insurance Service; 2015.
53. Kang IO, Park CY, Lee Y. Role of healthcare in Korean long-term care insurance. J Korean Med Sci. 2012;27:S41–6.
54. Oh YH, Lee YK, Sunwoo D, Yoo HY, Oh JS. Networking healthcare and social services for those outside the long-term care insurance. Sejong: Korea Institute for Health and Social Affairs; 2009.
55. Lee Y, Lim BW, Chang KO, Kim HY. Establishing the Gyeonggi Care Center for older people. Suwon: Ajou University; 2004.
56. Lee HK. Linking health and welfare services and the applications. Korean J Gerontol Soc Welfare. 2001;12:175–207.
57. Lee Y, Kim KH, Kim JL, Jeong PL. Evaluation of health and welfare linkage project for older adults in Suwon. Suwon: Ajou University; 2002.
58. Ministry of Health and Welfare. 2019 community security council operation manual. Sejong: Ministry of Health and Welfare; 2019.
59. Kim SY, Change IH, Kim JW, Kwon HY. Conceptualization and strategies for Korean community care by comparison with overseas cases. Seoul: The Seoul Institute; 2018.
60. Hwang GY. The outreach community centers initiative: policy recommendations for improvement. Health Welfare Policy Forum. 2017;11:21–41.
61. Lee KS, Sagong J, Han MK, Park YM. Community care: theory and policy. Seoul: Korea Institute for Health and Welfare Policy; 2019.

Chapter 2
The United States Perspective on Community-Based Integrated Care

Cheryl Phillips

What Is "Integrated, Community-Based Care?"

Integrated care refers to the bringing together of inputs, delivery, management, and organization of services as a means of improving access, quality, patient satisfaction, and efficiency. This concept was originally introduced as a vision of how health care organizations and health systems should address the changing demands of society. Community-based integrated care can also function as a concrete strategy to synergistically embed all quality improvement efforts within our health systems. It creates various rationalization strategies that can be combined by taking the reduction of fragmentation in health care delivery and a consistent focus on the health of the community as a starting point. Of course, these efforts at integration are still working within an existing system built on specialization and a focus on disease-specific care. Many older people in the United States have multiple comorbidities and many medical appointments.

Integrated care may be seen as a response to the fragmented delivery of health and social services, which is an acknowledged problem in many health systems. The continuity of care is closely related to integrated care and emphasizes the patient's perspective through the system of health and social services, providing valuable lessons for the integration of systems. Three central themes in terms of working together effectively in an integrated model of care include autonomy, coordination, and integration (connecting with provider and health care workers in varying capacities and different settings and levels of care).

According to the World Health Organization (2002), "Integrated care is a concept bringing together inputs, delivery, management and organization of services

C. Phillips (✉)
SNP Alliance, Washington, DC, USA
e-mail: cphillips@snpalliance.org

M. K. McNabney (ed.), *Community-Based Integrated Care for Older Adults*,
https://doi.org/10.1007/978-3-031-05137-1_2

related to diagnosis, treatment, care, rehabilitation and health promotion. Integration is a means to improve services in relation to access, quality, user satisfaction and efficiency." Community-based care and services are those that are provided in the home (community) as opposed to health care facilities like nursing homes and hospitals.

What Makes Integrated Community-Based Care Teams Unique?

Community-based integrated care has been a cornerstone of care for older people in the United States for over half a century. In the mid-1980s, with the shifting focus on "chronic care," [1] the concept of "integration" emerged in the literature and in practice. Integrated care was often used to describe health care systems that had a horizontal alignment of practices and services and vertical connections between providers and services in a variety of settings [2]. Sadly, such "integrated" relationships often meant only contractual connections and a common letterhead for the parent organization. Even today, the term "integration" has many meanings. For behavioral health providers, it means the inclusion of mental health into mainstream medical care; for policy makers, it often means the operational linkage of US payers, such as Medicare and Medicaid; for health care systems, it may reflect horizontal and vertical business affiliations and acquisitions. For the purpose of this chapter, the definition of *integrated care* is person-centered care that is based on an individual needs assessment that incorporates and coordinates the person's medical and behavioral health, functional support, social support needs, and family/caregiver resources and coordinates information and services across providers and home and community-based services (HCBS) and is built on the person's goals and preferences.

But what does integrated care look like to the older individual receiving such services? First of all, most people already see their lives, however challenging, as already *integrated*. It is the fragmentation of disease-based US health care services; the distinction of physical, social, functional, and behavioral health needs and services; and the unaligned payment rules and eligibilities that create the *disintegrated* maze that many older Americans with complex needs must navigate. Thus, true integrated care requires the alignment of services and providers, regulations, health care policies and payment, and the actual systems of care delivery.

Community-based integrated care for older adults includes not only the complex interactions of comorbid chronic conditions, but it must also focus on functional support needs, behavioral health and cognition, history or the presence of substance use disorders, and individual person-centered goals and advance care wishes. It must take into account the varied structures of support systems—including available family, friends, and direct care providers (either paid or unpaid). It must acknowledge the environment in which the person lives, such as reliable and safe housing, transportation, access to nutritious and appropriate food, and the ability to manage medications. The integration of all these aspects of the older person's health and well-being requires a team and close connections with HCBS.

Community-based care teams in the United States have been evolving in the past several decades. The most studied and well known of these teams are the interdisciplinary teams (IDTs) within the Program of All-Inclusive Care for the Elderly (PACE) model. Other examples of team models studied in the United States include the Social Health Maintenance Organization (SHMO) model, which was discontinued in 2002 [3]; the Independence at Home Demonstration [4]; patient-centered medical homes [5]; and Indiana University's Grace model [6]. Each of these integrated community care teams creates a culture of interdependence with each other, with the community services, and with the individual at the center.

Early work with clinical care teams focused on the "multidisciplinary" nature of teamwork—where each discipline represented in the team contributed (often at different times and settings) to the care planning of the person. This concept evolved into the "interdisciplinary teams," where each discipline brought its own perspective into the team dialogue—but still focused on individual professional boundaries. The most successful community-based integrated care teams evolve into "transdisciplinary" teams—where the teams expand to include members without formal clinical licenses, such as transportation drivers, home care workers, community workers and coaches, and service coordinators from senior housing communities. While transdisciplinary does not mean that the scope of license and accountabilities disappear, it does mean that the conversation, centered on the person and their goals, takes input and direction across all voices. The van driver may observe a new, unrecognized, fall risk. The service coordinator may identify particular services available to the individual in the housing community, and the mental health liaison may share particular stressors the individual is experiencing.

Integrated care also means including the behavioral health needs and support and treatment of substance use disorders, when present. For the past several decades, primary care has sought to include behavior health in whole-person practice. The US Veterans Affairs (VA) established a full-time mental health provider in each VA home-based primary care team. They report that not only was this integration feasible, but it also resulted in a high degree of team interaction and practice and can also serve as a model of mental health care for home-bound and other older adults [7].

There are also "informal care systems" that are created by older adults, along with a network of family and friends who serve as caregivers, advisors, and transportation. These care teams are often not recognized and not sufficiently utilized to maximize benefits for the patient. For example, many aspects of care assessments and assistance with transitions are being done outside of the formal care teams discussed below. As a result, these informal care teams are typically not "integrated" within the system.

What Makes Community-Based Integrated Care Successful?

What tends to sustain these integrated approaches is a sense of trust between team members and a culture of team participation where each voice and contribution is valued and the outcome is greater than any discipline or person would develop. Kodner and Kyriacou outlined 15 operational characteristics integral to the development and operationalization of integrated care, which includes a funding mechanism, comprehensive service package and network connections, the ability to target at-risk populations and follow up individual assessments, information sharing, and the ability of the team to remain connected with primary care and with each other [8].

Clarity in purpose and process is also essential for the success of community-based integrated teams. The parent or sponsoring organization must embrace shared alignment and purpose that goes beyond mere cost containment. For example, a hospital system that relies on fee-for-service admissions for cardiac-related diagnoses may initially support an integrated community-based team that helps individuals self-manage their conditions and focuses on barriers that individuals may face when it comes to medication adherence, appropriate nutrition, or transportation for needed outpatient medical visits. But if that hospital system is only looking at economics, they may waiver in their support when admissions for this population decrease (hence resulting in revenue loss) or when the costs of supporting the team are equal to or greater than any cost savings the system realized (cost shifting). Ultimately, a shared value system and shared incentives are required to sustain an integrated community-based program. And with shared incentives, there must also be a clear understanding of who receives the benefits. While improved person-reported quality of life and reported health and well-being have been fairly constant outcomes of these models, sustaining them also requires measurable benefits to the supporting organization. This benefit can take many forms. It can mean that medical-surgical beds are available for (more lucrative) tertiary care and elective procedures. It may provide support for the system's stated community mission. It may be a source of outside fundraising. It may even be valued in the form of managing risk in alternative payment models. Most likely, the benefits to the parent system are any number of combinations of the above, and a truly successful integrated community-based model will understand, measure, and leverage these for continued support and success.

Who Pays for the Services?

While understanding the incentives for the parent organization is support the team is essential to sustain the program, determining who pays for the needed nonmedical services is far more challenging for most models. There is a myriad of community-based programs, including adult day care, Veterans Administration services, senior community center programs, and Older Americans Act meal programs, just to name a few. Each has its own eligibility criteria and payment sources. This quickly creates a maze that is virtually unnavigable by the individual and their families and is chaotic, at best, for the care team to coordinate. Medicaid does offer some support services, known as long-term services and supports (LTSS), but Medicaid eligibility and the scope of benefits vary from state to state. Furthermore, many LTSS services are referral based and have little linkage, or integration, with the primary care team.

Those dually eligible for both Medicare and Medicaid have a greater risk of needing support services than the average nondual beneficiary. The Medicare Payment Advisory Commission, in its 2018 report, noted that 30 percent of those dually eligible need assistance with three or more activities of daily living (ADLs) as compared to just 9% of the nondual Medicare beneficiaries [9]. This same report also stated that those dually eligible have Medicare per person per year costs two times as high as nondual Medicare beneficiaries, and often have more complex medical needs with comorbid chronic conditions. Historically, the two payment systems grew out of separate structures and eligibilities. Medicare was designed to address the medical care of all older Americans based on age alone, while Medicaid was created to address "social" needs based on low-income status and was so structured that states determine the eligibility criteria and scope of benefits. Recognizing that both medical and social services are intertwined for older adults with medical and functional support needs, new models of payment have emerged. The PACE program was the first and most comprehensive when it comes to integrating Medicare and Medicaid into one program and provided the scope of their services, which were based on individual needs.

In 2003, Congress approved and authorized **special needs plans (SNPs)**, and in 2018, they were made permanent. SNPs are a subset of managed Medicare, also known as Medicare Advantage (MA), and have specific enrollment criteria based on the SNP type. Chronic SNPs (C-SNPs) target those with serious and potentially life-threatening chronic conditions. Enrollees must have one of the 15 eligible chronic conditions, verified by the person's physician. Institutional (or I-SNPs) enroll those who are at a nursing home level of care, as determined by their state, for at least 90 days. While most do reside as long-stay residents of nursing homes, other plans have targeted assisted living, senior living communities, or other senior housing locations. Dually eligible SNPs (D-SNPs) enroll those who are dually eligible for Medicaid and Medicare. There are also two distinct subtypes of D-SNPs, namely, highly integrated dually eligible (HIDE) and fully integrated dually eligible (FIDE) SNPs. In a HIDE-SNP, although the enrollment may not be fully aligned, the parent organization of the D-SNP must also contract with the state for a managed LTSS plan, and the HIDE SNP must integrate LTSS and/or behavioral health services. A FIDE-SNP has a much higher degree of integration. The MA plan offering the D-SNP must also have a state Medicaid contract for LTSS. The FIDE-SNP must coordinate the delivery of covered Medicare and Medicaid services using aligned care management and specialty care network methods for high-risk beneficiaries. And the FIDE-SNP is also responsible for 180 days of nursing home coverage (Table 2.1). The focus of all D-SNPs is to attempt to integrate and coordinate both

Table 2.1 Basic criteria: FIDE-SNPs, HIDE-SNPs, and D-SNPs[a]

Requirement	FIDE-SNP	HIDE-SNP	D-SNP
Must have existing, executed contract(s) with the state Medicaid agency in the state(s) in which the entity seeks to operate by July 6, 2020 (for CY 2021)	Yes	Yes	Yes
Must have a contract with the state Medicaid agency that meets the requirements of a managed care organization as defined in section 1903(m) of the Social Security Act	Yes	No	No
Must have a capitated contract with the state Medicaid agency to provide coverage of long-term services and supports (LTSS), consistent with state policy	Yes The contract must be with the same MA organization	No The state Medicaid contract may be with 1. The MA organization offering the D-SNP 2. The MA organization's parent organization or 3. Another entity owned and controlled by the MA organization's parent organization	No
Must have a capitated contract with the state Medicaid agency to provide coverage of behavioral health services, consistent with state policy	No Complete carve out of behavioral health coverage by the state Medicaid agency is permitted	No (If it otherwise covers LTSS)	No
Must have a capitated contract with the state Medicaid agency to provide coverage of a minimum of 180 days of nursing facility services during the plan year	Yes	No	No
Must coordinate all services, including Medicaid fee for service grievance and appeals	Yes	Yes	Yes
Must specify a process to share information with the state Medicaid agency (or state's designee), on hospital and SNF admissions for at least one group of high-risk individuals who are enrolled in the D-SNP	No	No	Yes
Must agree to use the unified appeals and grievance procedures outlined in the rule if the D-SNP meets the definition for exclusively aligned enrollment[b]	Yes	Yes	No

Table 2.1 (continued)

Requirement	FIDE-SNP	HIDE-SNP	D-SNP
Must coordinate the delivery of covered Medicare and Medicaid services using aligned care management and specialty care network methods for high-risk beneficiaries	Yes	No	No
Must employ policies and procedures approved by CMS and the state to coordinate or integrate beneficiary communication materials, enrollment, communications, grievance and appeals, and quality improvement	Yes	No	No

[a] *FIDE* fully integrated dual eligible SNP, *HIDE* highly integrated dual eligible SNP, *D-SNP* dual eligible SNP

[b] Exclusively aligned enrollment is defined as the D-SNP that exclusively enrolls full-benefit dual eligible individuals whose Medicaid benefits are covered under a Medicaid managed care contract under section 1903(m) of the SSA between the applicable state and the SNP's MA organization, the SNP's parent organization, or another entity that is owned and controlled by the D-SNP's parent organization

Medicare and Medicaid benefits—most often through a managed Medicaid Long-Term Service and Supports (MLTSS) plan. As of April 2020, there are over 3.4 million individuals enrolled in special needs plans, with over 86% enrolled in D-SNPs (including HIDE- and FIDE-SNPs) [10].

SNPs have several requirements that serve to support an integrated team-based concept. Each SNP must have a Model of Care (MOC) created and approved by the National Committee for Quality Assurance (NCQA). This MOC must include the following elements of how the plan will provide care for the targeted population: a description of the SNP population; how care coordination will be provided, including how they will complete an initial and annual health risk appraisal and an individualized care plan; who is on the interdisciplinary team and how transitions of care will be managed; details of the SNP provider network; and quality measurement and performance improvement, including goal setting. While the operational details of this coordination are not included in SNP regulations, typically successful SNPs have community-based workers who meet directly with individuals and communicate with both health plan and primary care teams to address new issues and unmet service needs.

The Affordable Care Act, Section 2602, created the Federal Coordinated Health Care Office. One of the strategies of this office was to align the two public payment programs under the Federal Alignment Initiative – which included the Medicare-Medicaid demonstration plans (MMPs). The first demonstration began in 2013. These plans require a three-way contract between the Centers for Medicare and Medicaid (CMS), the state, and the health plan and also focus on those dually eligible. The Centers for Medicare and Medicaid (CMS) have published 11 evaluations to date. While the primary outcome for these evalutations was cost savings, care coordination that identified the individual's specific needs and coordinated available community services was seen as key to the programs' success [11].

What makes all these models, including PACE, financially viable? Each involves some measures of risk sharing and population-based financing. Under the traditional fee-for-service model, there needs to be the ability to bill directly the activities of the team members, as well as care coordination activities. Because the assumption is that integrated team-based models help reduce avoidable costs for targeted, high-risk individuals, population-based payments that involve risk sharing, rather than traditional fee for service, have the added flexibility of paying for such services—not as revenue centers but as opportunities to reduce costs and improve care [12].

The models described above are all "capitation" payment models, prepaid payments based on the number of enrolled people, or "per capita." However, risk sharing may be present in a variety of alternative payment models (APMs), including accountable care organizations (ACOs), medical homes, managed fee-for-service contracts, and even some direct-to-provider pilots and demonstrations proposed by the Center for Medicare and Medicaid Innovation (CMMI). How effectively these APMs utilize integrated teams is often dependent on their unique financing structure—who is taking the risk and who shares in the savings.

What Does the Future Hold?

As the definitions of health and well-being increasingly recognize the role of a person's living situation, finances, and social support (commonly defined as social determinants of health (SDOH)), the need for truly integrated teams will continue to grow. Community integrated teams can also serve to address these social determinates for older adults who often deal with complex medical needs, functional supports, social isolation, food and housing insecurity, and behavioral health issues. Successfully addressing social determinants requires community-based teams that can navigate community services and are skilled at person-centered goals and have a direct connection with the primary care team.

Key successes for this type of integration must, as its foundation, include person-centered goals and planning. Integration cannot just be a medical tool to reduce costs and improve outcomes. It must also be a tool for the individual to make their preferences known and to create a plan of care that truly reflects who they are and what they want. Team-based care can be a vehicle for such person centeredness as long as the person (or their care partners or family) is actually part of the "team." While there is some early work on person-centered planning, there is considerable learning and development needed for integrated teams to fully embrace this skill set.

Perhaps the greatest challenge in the immediate future is the lack of a skilled and trained workforce. The 2009 Institute of Medicine report, *Retooling for an Aging American: Building the Health Care* Workforce [13], acknowledges the challenge for those skilled in geriatric medicine and nursing, social work, mental health, pharmacy, and therapy and, more importantly, for direct care workers. In many ways, team-based care becomes a part of the workforce solution since the team approach can optimize the use of each of the member's skills and training.

Future Policy Direction

Expanding access to community-based integrated care in the U.S. wil require addressing many current regulatory barriers: health plan enrollment reqirments to align both Medicare and Medicaid; quality measures that focus on *outcomes* for individuals with complex needs; shared-savings that align incentives for payers, provider and those receiving care; and assistance for health plans and state Medicaid offices to partner with community organization and services.

Integration is the bringing together of the whole-person needs. It requires coordination of payment, policy, and delivery systems. It relies on shared information and technology to serve as a tool to enhance that exchange of information. It is built on a *transdisciplinary* team that is part of the community, that can navigate resources and services, and that is also connected to the medical care and primary care team. Most importantly, it is not "for" the person served nor "about" the person—but "with" the individual as they direct interventions that reflect their own preferences and goals. US policy makers continue to focus on strategies to better integrate Medicare and Medicaid, as well as identify models that focus on the whole-person needs across settings and services to reduce avoidable costs and improve the quality of care.

References

1. Wagner EH, Austin BT, Von Korff D. Organizing care for patients with chronic illness. Millbank Q. 1996;74(4):511–44.
2. Kodner DL, Spreeuwenberg C. Integrated care: meaning, logic, applications, and implications—a discussion paper. Int J Integr Care. 2002;2:e12.
3. Tompson, T. Evaluation Results for the Social/Health Maintenance Organization II Demonstration, Secretary of Health and Human Services Report to Congress, 2002. https://innovation.cms.gov/files/migrated-medicare-demonstration-x/shmo_report.pdf. Accessed 17 April 2020.
4. Centers for Medicare and Medicaid. Independence at Home Fact Sheet; 2019. https://innovation.cms.gov/files/fact-sheet/iah-fs.pdf. Accessed 17 April 2020.
5. Epperly T. The patient-centered medical home in the USA. J Eval Clin Pract. 2011;17:373–5.
6. Bielaszka-DuVernay C. The "grace model": in-home assessments lead to better care for dual eligible. Health Aff. 2011;30(3):431–4.
7. Karlin B, Karel M. National integration of mental health provider in VA home-based primary care: an innovative model for mental health care delivery with older adults. The Gerontologist. 2013;54(5):868–79.
8. Kodner D, Kyriacou C. Fully integrated care for frail elderly: two American models. Int J Integr Care. 2000;1:1.

9. Medicare Payment Advisory Commission and Medicaid and CHIP Payment and Access Commission Data Book, Beneficiaries Dually Eligible for Medicare and Medicaid. 2018. http://medpac.gov/docs/default-source/data-book/jan18_medpac_macpac_dualsdatabook_sec.pdf?sfvrsn=0%20%20. Accessed 18 April 2020.
10. Plochg T, Ilinca S, Noordegraaf M. Beyond integrated care. J Health Serv Res Policy. 2017;23:195–7.
11. Centers for Medicare and Medicaid SNP Comprehensive Report. 2020. https://www.cms.gov/research-statistics-data-and-systemsstatistics-trends-and-reportsmcradvpartdenroldataspecial-needs/snp-comprehensive-report-2020-04. Accessed 18 April 2020.
12. Centers for Medicare and Medicaid. Evaluations of integrated care models for dually eligible beneficiaries: key findings and research gaps. 2019. https://www.cms.gov/Medicare-Medicaid-Coordination/Medicare-and-Medicaid-Coordination/Medicare-Medicaid-Coordination-Office/FinancialAlignmentInitiative/Evaluations.html. Accessed 23 May 2020.
13. The Institute of Medicine of the National Academies. Retooling for an aging America building the health care workforce. Washington, D.C., 2008.

Part II
The U.S. Prototype: Program of All-Inclusive Care for the Elderly (PACE)

Chapter 3
History and Policy Evolution of the PACE Model of Care

Shawn Bloom

The PACE Model of Care

The Program of All-Inclusive Care for the Elderly (PACE) is a well-established care delivery and financing model for older adults over age 55 whose level of care needs is deemed to be equivalent to that of people living in nursing homes. In 2021, there were 140 PACE organizations in 30 states, with enrollments ranging from about 50 to over 3000 participants per program. **Ninety percent of PACE participants are "dually eligible" for Medicare and Medicaid, 9% are eligible only for Medicaid, and less than 1% are eligible only for Medicare**.

PACE organizations (POs) serve those people who are among the most vulnerable of Medicare and Medicaid recipients—adults over age 55 who are assessed and certified by their state as meeting their state's definition of needing a nursing home level of care. Participants typically have multiple, complex medical conditions as well as functional and/or cognitive impairments. Fully integrated PACE organizations provide program participants with all needed medical and supportive services, including the entire continuum of Medicare- and Medicaid-covered items and services, with the objective of maintaining the independence of participants in their homes and communities for as long as possible.

The hallmark of the PACE model is an interdisciplinary team (IDT) made up of primary care providers, nurses, social workers, physical, occupational and recreational therapists, and numerous other health care professionals. All members of the IDT are directly employed by the PO, with a few exceptions. This IDT comprehensively assesses participants' care needs and develops and implements participant-centered care plans. Services are provided by the staff in the

S. Bloom (✉)
National PACE Association, Alexandria, VA, USA
e-mail: shawnb@npaonline.org

M. K. McNabney (ed.), *Community-Based Integrated Care for Older Adults*,
https://doi.org/10.1007/978-3-031-05137-1_3

PACE center, a unique setting that combines the attributes of a primary care clinic, adult day health care center, and physical therapy and occupational therapy clinic (see Chaps. 9 and 19). Services are also provided in participants' homes and, when necessary, in inpatient settings.

Services include, but are not limited to, the following:

- Adult day care, which offers nursing; physical, occupational, and recreational therapies; meals; nutritional counseling; social work; and personal care
- Medical care provided by a PACE physician, nurse practitioner, or physician assistant who is familiar with the history, needs, and preferences of each participant
- Home health care and personal care
- All necessary prescription drugs
- Social services
- Medical specialties, such as audiology, dentistry, optometry, podiatry, and speech therapy
- Respite care; and
- Hospital and nursing home care, when necessary

Although all PACE participants are certified as clinically eligible to receive nursing home care by their state, few are residing or receiving care in a facility; only about 5% of PACE participants actually reside in a nursing home. This low percentage is achieved despite the fact that, on average, PACE participants have six chronic conditions (including 46% who have dementia and over 40% who have a serious mental illness).

With respect to payment, the mean Medicaid capitation rate in 2020 paid by states to PACE organizations for each PACE participant was $3981, and the mean Medicare capitated payment was $2797, with no service limitations, copays, or deductibles (NPA Annual PACE Capitation Rate Survey, June 2020). Capitated payments for all Medicare and Medicaid services align PACE organizations' financial incentives with the quality of care their participants seek. Under this capitated arrangement, PACE organizations are incentivized to keep participants as well as possible in order to reduce inpatient hospital and skilled nursing facility costs. Evidence shows PACE organizations generally have lower inpatient hospital use and shorter hospital lengths of stay than comparable, non-PACE populations.

To achieve these desired outcomes, PACE IDTs work together to assess PACE participants' individualized needs, develop care plans, and provide and coordinate all primary, acute, and behavioral health and long-term services and supports (LTSS). The IDTs meet daily to discuss the emerging and ongoing care needs of the individuals for whom they are responsible. While people can literally see the PACE center and PACE vans, it is the PACE IDT that serves as the focal point of the PACE model of care and plays a vital role in the outcomes achieved.

Once enrolled, nearly all PACE participants remain in the program through the end of life, unless they move out of the geographic service area. In a 2018 survey of

973 caregivers of PACE participants conducted by the National PACE Association, 96% of caregivers reported overall satisfaction with the services and 97% said they would recommend PACE to a family member in a similar situation.

History of On Lok and PACE

On Lok (Cantonese for "peaceful and happy abode") began its efforts to develop the PACE model of care in 1971 with an idea: traditional models of care in San Francisco were not meeting the needs of the elderly. Seniors wanted to age at home, but they needed services to maintain their independence. **Dr. William L. Gee and social worker Marie-Louise Ansak joined forces to create a program that would enable older adults to continue living in their community. Propelled by their drive and vision, On Lok founded the Program of All-Inclusive Care for the Elderly (PACE)** (NPA Caregiver Survey 2018).

On Lok Senior Health Services, a not-for-profit organization, was launched in the early 1970s in the Chinatown-North Beach area of San Francisco, California. With research and demonstration funding from the US Administration on Aging, On Lok opened an adult day health center in 1972, modeled on the British day hospital program.

In 1978, it expanded the model to include complete medical care and social support for the frail elderly and received federal waivers in 1979, which allowed reimbursement from Medicare for all outpatient health and health-related services. In 1980, inpatient services were added, including skilled nursing care and acute hospitalization. In 1983, amendments to the Social Security Act provided that On Lok be given authority to test a risk-based financing system involving Medicare, Medicaid, and private pay. Major grants from the Robert Wood Johnson Foundation, the John A. Hartford Foundation, and the Retirement Research Foundation underwrote research and development activities to support this demonstration.

Congress extended On Lok's waivers indefinitely (1985) and provided waivers for the replication of the model at ten sites (1986). Through further support from the Robert Wood Johnson Foundation, On Lok provided technical assistance to help new sites develop and to create a cross-site database to track performance. **In 1990, the first replication sites received Medicare and Medicaid waivers as demonstration programs, and the model became known as the "Program of All-Inclusive Care for the Elderly" (PACE)**.

Various evaluations of the effectiveness of PACE have been conducted, which have yielded similar findings. One of the earliest studies by Abt Associates published in July of 1998 determined that "PACE was found to be associated with long-lasting decreases in nurse visits to the home, inpatient hospital admissions, inpatient hospital days, and nursing home days. The program also had a persistent, positive effect on ambulatory care visits and frequent attendance at social activities. PACE was associated with short-run improvements in quality of life, satisfaction with care, and functional status. Compared to individuals who were evaluated, accepted but declined PACE enrollment, PACE participants lived longer and spent more days in the community."

PACE Federal Policy Milestones

Permanent Provider Status

With the positive findings of the Abt study, On Lok facilitated the establishment of the National PACE Association (NPA) in 1994, which was comprised of the original 13 PACE demonstration programs. The original aim of the NPA was to advocate for Congressional recognition of PACE as a permanent Medicare benefit and an optional Medicaid state plan option. Working together, the members and staff of the NPA successfully accomplished this goal when the Balanced Budget Act of 1997 (BBA97) (P.L. 105-33, Sections 4801–4804) established PACE as a permanent part of the Medicare program and an option under state Medicaid programs.

In December 1999, the Centers for Medicare & Medicaid Services (CMS) issued the PACE final regulation, which has served as the basis for how PACE POs were required to operate and be accountable as fully integrated health care organizations entrusted with caring for frail older adults. The final rule provided an avenue for PACE demonstration organizations to transition to permanent provider status. After the completion of a comprehensive application process involving states and CMS, existing PACE demonstration programs became permanent PACE providers by 2003.

Benefit Improvement and Protection Act of 2000 PACE Waivers

Section 903 of the Benefits Improvement and Protection Act (BIPA) of 2000 allowed states to modify or waive certain regulatory provisions to meet the needs of PACE organizations (POs). The Centers for Medicare & Medicaid Services (CMS) has provided additional guidance on submitting waiver requests in the PACE program. The following provisions may not be waived:

- Focus on frail elderly qualifying individuals who require the level of care provided in a nursing facility
- Delivery of comprehensive, integrated acute and long-term care services
- Interdisciplinary team approach to care management and service delivery
- Capitated, integrated financing that allows the provider to pool payments received from public and private programs and individuals
- Assumption by the provider of full financial risks

The Benefits Improvement and Protection Act authorized CMS to waive certain PACE regulatory requirements. Section 902 grants the CMS Secretary the authority to grandfather operational modifications implemented by the initial 15 PACE demonstration programs. Specifically, the provision allows the PACE demonstrations to continue using program modifications, including the use of community-based providers (CBPs), that were in effect on July 1, 2000. PACE organizations using CBPs under BIPA 902 authority have "general organizational-wide waivers" that are permanent and do not need to be reviewed annually by CMS. Other PACE organizations that utilized CBPs as of July 1, 2000, were able to use CBPs as a result of Section 903 of BIPA. Section 903 granted CMS flexibility in exercising waiver authority provided under Sections 1894(f)(2)(B) and 1934(f)(2)(B) of the Social Security Act. Moreover, Section 903 allowed for specific modifications or waivers of certain regulatory provisions to meet the needs of PACE organizations, allowing them to utilize CBPs with the approval of CMS. PACE organizations that receive CBP waivers under Section 903 obtain "conditional organization-wide waivers," which require regular CMS assessments on the quality of care provided through the CBPs. In 2002, CMS established a process to submit and approve waiver requests, many of which are for CBPs.

Medicare Part D Prescription Drug Benefit

In 2003, the Medicare Modernization Act was passed and went into effect in 2006. This prescription drug benefit was an optional US federal government program to help Medicare beneficiaries pay for self-administered prescription drugs. This Medicare benefit had a significant impact on PACE program operations and is discussed in detail in Chap. 8.

Rural PACE Pilot Act

The need for PACE services in rural areas has long been recognized; however, the initial development of programs in urban areas reflects the greater population density and the greater availability of financial and service resources. While urban PACE programs have faced difficulties at start-up even in urban areas where health and funding resources were more readily available, these difficulties were considerably less than those that were anticipated in rural areas. In rural areas, where experience with PACE is extremely limited and the low density of the population raises greater concerns regarding the speed with which program census can grow, the requirement is a significant impediment to program growth.

In 2005, Congress established the Rural PACE (Program of All-Inclusive Care for the Elderly) Pilot Act to develop PACE as a noninstitutional option for frail rural elders. Today, 11 of the 15 pilot programs operate successfully across ten states, and nine more rural programs were established in recent years. With the "graying" of rural America, rural labor shortages, and limited noninstitutional long-term services and supports, plus a few innovative modifications, PACE has proved rural to be an effective care model supporting rural frail elders' desire to remain at home.

Rather than requiring that demonstration providers assume full financial risks from the onset of operations, the demonstration would afford them some protection in the first 3 years of program operations. Beyond that, it was hypothesized that the programs would achieve census levels adequate to sustain ongoing program operations without the protection afforded by risk sharing. In the first 3 years, however, Medicare would reimburse demonstration programs for some costs in excess of capitated revenues. In all instances, the program would share in these costs, thereby preserving the incentive to maximize efficiencies to the greatest extent possible. Further, the programs assumed progressively more risks over the course of the initial 3-year demonstration, and under no circumstances would Medicare assume risks for costs in excess of 25% of capitated payments.

Another critical component of the demonstration's risk-sharing approach is that programs would be required to set aside any surplus revenue in a risk reserve that would be allocated in the event of subsequent years' program losses or allocated to program enhancements, such as additional personnel, equipment, or space, or to the repayment of debt incurred with respect to program start-up, except where within 30 days of notice of the proposed use the Secretary specifically disapproves. To the extent that any risk reserves exceed twice the sum of 3 months' costs at the conclusion of the initial 3-year demonstration period, any difference will be returned to Medicare.

This approach to risk sharing achieves three principal objectives: (1) it affords demonstration providers some financial protection initially and encourages their participation in the demonstration, (2) it addresses the financial consequences of both slow census growth and the possibility of enrolling one or more participants that may experience a catastrophic event that would generate high costs to the program before there is a sufficient number of enrollees across which to spread such costs, and (3) it limits Medicare's financial exposure to not more than it would have had if the program's enrollees remained in fee-for-service Medicare.

The legislation supported the establishment of 13 rural PACE organizations, which received grants of $800,000 to support development and start-up costs. NPA supported their development efforts by providing training and ongoing technical assistance over a 2-year period. Today, ten of the original 13 rural programs remain operational and have provided a framework for the establishment of rural PACE, which has enabled many other programs to be developed in nonurban areas of the country.

Strategic Efforts to Support the Expansion of PACE

PACE Expansion Initiative (PEI)

In 2000, the NPA board of directors recognized the need to support the establishment and expansion of PACE across the country. Building on the generous and historical support of the John A. Hartford Foundation (JAHF) and the Robert

Wood Johnson Foundation (JAHF), the association secured funding to pursue the goal of expanding access to PACE. To achieve this goal, the PACE Expansion Initiative (PEI) focused on four critical constituencies: federal and state policy makers, providers, and consumers, including potential PACE enrollees and their caregivers.

The proposed activities for this project were organized into the following three areas of focus: federal regulatory and legislative activities, expanding provider capacity, state policy activities, and enhancing awareness of PACE.

Expanding Provider Capacity

The primary objective of activities in this area was to expand the number of providers that elect to pursue PACE development by expanding very substantially the resources available to providers to implement PACE. First, due to the complex nature of the PACE program, which is simultaneously a managed care entity, direct service provider, and Medicare and Medicaid contractor, **there was a heightened need for technical assistance** in navigating the intricate set of operational and regulatory requirements imposed on PACE. Typically, prospective providers and their staff have strength in providing either acute or long-term care services but not both. For those who come from an acute care perspective, the Medicaid and long-term care aspects of the program are more challenging. For those with a long-term care background, Medicare and particularly Medicare managed care and all it entails presented a greater obstacle. **The ability of NPA to fill the knowledge gap in these areas could contribute to a more efficient start-up**. It will help in persuading organizations weighing the costs of PACE start-up in terms of time and resources to move forward.

Development and Dissemination of Written Products

NPA staff had experience in analyzing regulatory issues and their impact on PACE from the public policy perspective. However, NPA had been less effective in assisting prospective providers and existing NPA members to respond efficiently to regulatory and operational requirements. Consequently, each organization that was actively assessing the costs and benefits of becoming a PACE provider included in that calculation significant expenditures, in terms of both time and money, to develop systems, materials, etc. As such NPA proposed to develop these materials as model practice templates fine-tuned the resources by experienced PACE providers. The following are examples of such products:

- PACE program model policies and procedures to provide prospective providers a detailed understanding of program operations as well as boilerplate language for their PACE provider applications, e.g., policies and procedures for enrollment and disenrollment, grievances and appeals, credentialing

- Model contracts between PACE organizations and key contract providers, e.g., hospitals, nursing homes, and medical specialists, that are consistent with PACE and applicable Medicare+Choice (now Medicare Advantage) regulatory requirements
- Model marketing materials, including an Enrollee Handbook and a marketing plan that meet federal requirements
- Model Bill of Participant Rights
- Model Quality Assessment and Performance Improvement Plan
- Model Compliance Plan
- Model job descriptions for key PACE personnel; and
- Handbook on encounter reporting requirements, including a "Super Bill" designed specifically for PACE programs identifying the most common diagnoses and procedures for PACE enrollees

NPA provided the materials developed under this project to NPA members as a benefit for their membership, the dues for which, at the time, ranged from $3500 to $20,000 for provider entities. The dissemination of these products was intended to enhance providers' interest in PACE and contribute to the efficient and consistent development of the PACE model. Further, by making these products available as a benefit of NPA membership, the incentive to join NPA will increase significantly, thereby further enhancing NPA's ability to sustain these activities on an ongoing basis.

Development and Implementation of Training Sessions and Accompanying Materials

In addition to the written products identified above, educational sessions and audio-conferences were effective strategies for conveying information on regulatory and operational requirements. NPA organized focused training sessions and accompanying technical assistance materials on a variety of topics. Examples of topics offered included the PACE provider application, compliance with the financial reporting standards of the National Association of Insurance Commissioners, effective marketing strategies for PACE, and physician-and-outpatient-encounter reporting. The objective of the training sessions was to provide attendees with the information they need to respond to requirements in an efficient manner. Relative to larger providers or Medicare+Choice plans, the resources available to PACE organizations to address these requirements were limited, if not nonexistent. Efforts to streamline activities in response to their requirements supported existing sites enormously and lessened deterrents to pursuing PACE development in the first place.

NPA also offered training for PACE primary care physicians and nurse practitioners on clinical leadership in PACE. Recognizing that the strength of the primary care practitioner in PACE is a major factor in the program's overall success, NPA worked with its Primary Care Committee to identify a Master Clinicians Panel to develop the session, including a curriculum, training objectives, and a syllabus of published and unpublished resources. Broadly, the session reviewed the critical role and responsibilities of the primary care practitioner in PACE, both individually and vis-à-vis the PACE interdisciplinary team.

Specialized Technical Assistance

In addition to providing standardized materials and in-depth training, project staff provided individualized technical assistance to interested organizations. A key aspect of this project was to market NPA as a source of technical assistance for organizations considering PACE development. This was done primarily through NPA's website, phone consultation, and other dissemination activities, which are listed below in the section titled "Enhancing Awareness of PACE." In addition, if an organization sought on-site technical assistance from NPA, some percentage of project staff time would be available for this (travel expenses would be incurred by the organization seeking technical assistance).

NPA partnered with the PACE Technical Assistance Centers (TACs) to assist potential PACE sponsors with start-up assistance, training, and other forms of support. Under the original PACE demonstration, On Lok, the original PACE TAC, and subsequently other demonstration sites developed a capacity to provide technical assistance to organizations considering PACE development. The TACs are typically engaged by organizations exploring the possibility of developing PACE to undertake a feasibility assessment that focuses on five critical areas:

1. Analysis of the potential demand for PACE services within the geographic catchment area identified by the organization
2. Analysis of how a PACE program will complement and/or compete with the organization's existing programs and consideration of how the PACE program should fit into the organization's administrative structure and service delivery system(s)
3. Analysis of the state's long-term care system and consideration of how PACE might fit within that system and, to varying degrees depending on the specifics of the situation, participation in conversations between the prospective PACE provider and the state on a variety of key development and implementation issues, e.g., Medicaid rate setting, licensing, contracting
4. Development of a 5-year budget based on assumptions drawn from the existing experience of PACE programs, e.g., utilization rates, staffing patterns; and
5. Development of a work plan to accompany the budget, which spans a 5-year period, including 1 year for development, prior to the initiation of program operations

State Policy Activities

The role of states in expanding PACE cannot be overstated. Unless a state chooses to develop PACE as a voluntary option under its Medicaid program, the prospects for PACE within that state are poor. **The success of the PACE model can be attributed largely to a good working relationship that has evolved between states and provider organizations**. Project staff focused on state activities that would both plan and execute multistate activities and respond to individual states' requests for specific information related to program development, implementation, and expansion. In this area, NPA project staff:

- Acted as a clearinghouse for states for both information on PACE and contacts in other states who could be resources to them.
- Built on the resources developed with funding from the Retirement Research Foundation to convene a State Work Group, which yielded four issues briefs that address a variety of PACE development and implementation issues from the perspective of states, e.g., provider selection, rate setting, contracting, licensing. This project would provide NPA with resources to work individually with states to interpret the issue briefs in states' unique long-term care environments.
- Developed additional written resources that approach PACE issues from states' perspectives, e.g., Responses to Frequently Asked Questions.
- Expanded NPA's support for hosting an annual meeting addressing State Contacts on PACE.

Expanding Awareness of PACE Among Consumers, Providers, and Policy Makers

An important element in expanding the PACE model and the number of individuals served by PACE under the project was to enhance awareness of the program and its benefits among health care providers; state policy makers, who ultimately determine whether PACE is developed within their states; and consumers. Because the number of PACE sites was limited under the demonstration to not more than 15, PACE had not been viewed as an option with broad-scale applicability. As such, it was important to educate key constituencies about PACE and the program's new status as a permanent provider under Medicare and Medicaid state options. A marketing campaign targeting health care entities and state policy makers, encouraging them to consider PACE development, and potential consumers of PACE services, informing them of the benefits of PACE, proved critical to achieving this project's objective of expanding PACE.

Examples of strategies NPA employed to expand awareness included the following:

1. *For health care providers*—with the objective of stimulating greater levels of provider interest in PACE development by presenting the merits of PACE vis-à-vis other opportunities that health care organizations may be considering for future growth and/or expansion:

a. Develop and submit articles for publication in appropriate journals and trade association publications explaining the PACE program and its benefits from the perspective of organizations that would be likely to consider PACE development, e.g., hospital systems and institutional and community-based long-term care providers.
b. Develop a slide presentation for delivery at allied trade association conferences, in response to specific requests by individual health care organizations, and other venues designed to inform providers about PACE and engage them to consider PACE development.
c. Develop a packet of materials for targeted mailing to health care organizations and posting on NPA's website summarizing the PACE model and the PACE developmental process. Identify the NPA as a resource for entities that would like to follow up regarding the receipt of these materials and provide technical assistance to them as required.

2. *For state policymakers* – with the objective of expanding the number of states that elect to develop PACE as a Medicaid state option and expanding the limited number of sites within states where PACE already exists:

   a. Develop and submit articles for publication in journals and other publications read by state policy makers in an effort to heighten awareness of PACE as a high-quality, cost-effective option that states can incorporate into their long-term care systems.
   b. Develop a slide presentation for delivery at state conferences, state meetings focused on the integration of Medicare and Medicaid services for dual eligibles, etc., explaining the PACE model where it fits within states' long-term care and managed care systems and identifying its pros and cons relative to other options that states may have for addressing the needs of dual eligibles.
   c. Establish contacts with state associations, e.g., the National Governors Association and the National Conference of State Legislatures, to educate staff about PACE.
   d. Target states that, to date, have not expressed interest in PACE and make information and resources available to them. In instances where NPA is aware of a prospective provider in these states, offer technical assistance in working with the state to evaluate the benefits and costs of PACE development.
   e. Expand the section of NPA's website dedicated to states to better address their needs.

3. *For consumers*—with the objective of understanding the elements of PACE that they find most and least attractive; this information would be used to develop model marketing materials for use by PACE programs and to identify needs for program innovation, which would respond to consumer preferences:

   a. Conduct market study and focus groups to identify the level of understanding and perceptions of PACE among consumers.

b. Test messages and marketing materials to promote a higher awareness and positive image of PACE as a desirable model of care for the frail elderly, particularly the middle income.
c. Identify family case studies that illustrate the benefits of PACE for use in marketing materials.
d. Develop and submit articles for publication in consumer publications.
e. Develop a slide presentation for delivery at conferences sponsored by consumer groups.
f. Establish contacts with key consumer groups, e.g., the American Association of Retired Persons (AARP).
g. Create model marketing materials for use by PACE sites based on the focus groups and messages identified to be effective in capturing the benefits of PACE.
h. Expand NPA's website to address consumer needs.

The PEI project proved successful in not only spawning interest in PACE expansion among states and prospective providers, but it also provided NPA with the resources and competencies to continue to support PACE growth and expansion. As interested organizations joined NPA for support, advocacy, and operational resources, dues revenue continued to grow providing NPA with revenues needed to sustain and build upon its ability to support PACE expansion. Lastly, PEI served as the platform for a long-term sustained effort by NPA to expand access to PACE.

Accelerating Access to PACE (ASAP)

NPA's initial efforts under PEI underscored the significant challenges state agencies face as essential partners with providers in expanding PACE services. The BBA requires that all PACE provider sites have the support of their state's administering agency for Medicaid-eligible seniors' health (usually the Medicaid agency but in some states the Department on Aging). To offer PACE, states must review and assess each provider's application, modify the Medicaid state plans they submit to the Health Care Financing Administration (HCFA) in order to receive federal matching funds, and put new systems in place to administer the program (financial, management, regulatory, and oversight). Further, state agencies must understand the nature of PACE sufficiently to implement financial, administrative, and oversight procedures to administer it as a Medicaid benefit. States are grappling with these issues in the context of an untested federal approach to PACE provider applications, efforts to apply aspects of Medicare managed care regulations to PACE providers, and HCFA's evolving oversight role relative to states.

Unless they were addressed, these challenges would delay and limit the ability to offer PACE to a greater number of frail elderly in a greater number of states (currently only 13 states have PACE sites). The first meeting of the Program Advisory Committee for PEI, held in March 2001, highlighted the significant barrier that delays in state action pose to new PACE services. Further, these delays raise potential PACE provider concerns about the risk of developing a PACE program, given the costs of investment and the extended time lag a site can face waiting to be operational.

Moreover, new PACE states that are poorly prepared to address issues such as rate setting and eligibility determination for PACE would place potential PACE providers at risk of making faulty, and financially significant, assumptions about these key factors in their financial model. Further, discussions by participants in the PACE State Workgroup meeting, a forum sponsored by the association for state administrators of current PACE programs to work with one another and with HCFA, emphasized the challenges that states face in implementing PACE. Indeed, the forum noted the challenges that even existing states face in interpreting and complying with recently issued HCFA regulations. The difficulties are all the more daunting to states in more preliminary stages of PACE development. Fundamentally, just as the ability of a PACE provider to initiate services and be successful depends on its state's support for PACE, the ability of NPA's efforts under PEI to increase PACE services nationally depends on our success in accelerating states' commitment to PACE and readiness to administer it.

Left unaddressed, the time delay caused by the barriers faced by states will lead many prospective PACE sites to reject PACE out of fear that their investment in PACE could "wither on the vine." Thus, PACE providers may find themselves facing mounting debts related to payroll and marketing costs because their states are not aggressively supporting enrollment in PACE, which is central to establishing adequate capitation revenues. State readiness to work with and support new providers, and to administer PACE as a benefit, is fundamental to the success of PEI and to the association's general goal of expanding PACE services for frail elders.

Even as states weighed the challenges of implementing a PACE benefit, the necessity of developing community-based alternatives to institutional care was compelling at the time. The Supreme Court decision on the *Olmstead* case found that institutionalizing individuals with disabilities who could be cared for in the community constituted discrimination under the Americans with Disabilities Act (ADA). In response, states were urgently looking for community-based alternatives to nursing home care. PACE provided a proven model for maintaining the frail elderly in the community. While the increased need for states to address community care provided an impetus for their adoption of PACE, the challenges of administering a PACE program seemed daunting, especially in light of states' need to simultaneously develop multiple PACE sites in order to provide broad coverage of their population.

Through the proposed ASAP project, the association was able to proactively identify and seek out states that have identified PACE as a priority in meeting their responsibility to provide community-based care for the frail elderly and that have a high likelihood of successful PACE implementation. The association worked with organizations such as the National Governors Association (NGA) as a partner in this process. The association undertook significant efforts to approach the selected states in partnership with it, through the provision of staff and training resources needed to expedite their successful start-up and the administration of a new PACE benefit, to successfully support states with expanded start-ups of new PACE organizations.

Rural PACE: Meeting the Challenge

The Deficit Reduction Act (DRA) of 2005 authorized a Rural PACE initiative, and in 2006, the Centers for Medicare and Medicaid Services (CMS) announced 15 rural PACE grantees. In 2006, the Department of Health and Human Services created the Rural PACE Provider Grant Program, which provided up to 15 grantees with $500,000 each to support the development of a rural PACE program. The National PACE Association and the National Rural Health Association (NRHA) received a contract from the Department to create a Rural PACE Technical Assistance Program, which produced resources for and provided technical assistance to organizations interested in developing a PACE program to serve a rural area.

Thanks to the legacy of that grant, **15% of existing PACE organizations exclusively serve rural communities**. In addition, many of the innovations that make PACE possible in rural communities are being considered innovations that might also improve the urban model or provide inspiration for how the PACE model could serve other high-need, high-cost individuals in the future.

As PACE programs expanded to rural communities, they adapted the model to better serve enrollees. In the traditional PACE model, a new enrollee would need to give up his/her physician and other providers and be solely served by the PACE IDT and the PACE network of specialists. However, approximately 40% of rural PACE organizations work with community physicians (providers who are outside the PACE IDT). By contracting with community physicians for primary care, PACE programs allow enrollees to preserve community relationships, thereby providing a way for enrollees to access services across a large geographical area.

Compared to urban-based PACE organizations, rural PACE organizations' service areas can be very large, often encompassing several communities and spanning several hundred square meters. Encouraging daily attendance in a central PACE center is not as feasible as in smaller service areas.

Another practice adopted by rural POs is to have several members of the IDT travel together to conduct home visits several days a week. In Colorado, one program shares an adult day center with non-PACE providers so that PACE services can be provided a few days a week at a location closer and more convenient than one of the existing PACE centers. In many instances, PACE organizations have used their position as a consumer of services in the community as a way to enhance or develop services for the entire community.

In Colorado, Senior CommUnity Care contracts for most of its transportation. However, it took it as a challenge to develop its services so it would serve the participants' needs. It developed new routes to accommodate where participants lived in their rural communities.

In Virginia, All Care contracted with a food service provider. The contract allowed the provider to expand its kitchen and the reach of its home-delivered meal services. The presence of the PACE program enabled that service to expand since the provider knew it had a reliable and regular customer.

PACE programs continue to grow and innovate in both rural and urban communities around the nation. PACE excels in serving some of the nation's most vulnerable populations and is ever striving toward keeping the elderly in their homes and communities.

PACE 2.0: Adapting and Disseminating PACE to Serve High-Need, High-Cost Populations

The Program of All-Inclusive Care for the Elderly (PACE) serves one of the most challenging high-need, high-cost populations – low-income, frail, older adults. PACE provides these older adults with an age-friendly health system that supports their ability to live at home, have their care needs met, and enjoy a high quality of life. **The recent enactment of the PACE Innovation Act allows for PACE to serve a wider range of high-need, high-cost adults through one or more pilots.**

For example, in addition to low-income, frail, older adults, PACE could serve people with physical, intellectual, or developmental disabilities; severe and persistent mental illness; or end-stage renal disease. While the legislation authorized payments to PACE pilot organizations for service delivery, it did not fund the development of PACE model adaptations for new populations or dissemination strategies related to these new opportunities. The development of these adaptations and strategies, combined with increased operational flexibility proposed by federal regulators, is required to set the stage for an exponential, rather than linear, rate of PACE growth.

With the goal of supporting PACE's exponential growth from 40,000 to 200,000 individuals, the National PACE Association created the PACE 2.0 project, which pursued a plan for adapted PACE models to serve a wider range of adults with high needs and high costs, including, but not limited to, PACE's current focus population of low-income, frail older adults.

Extending PACE 2.0 services requires adapting the care model's essential strengths to (1) meet the unique needs of different high-need, high-cost subpopulations and (2) support accelerated growth and access. The PACE 2.0 project provides the foundation for achieving these goals. By evaluating a high-need, high-cost subpopulation, the project estimated the number of people an adapted and more broadly disseminated PACE 2.0 model could serve. Using this estimate, the project will develop dissemination strategies for achieving exponential growth in PACE 2.0 services across a range of scenarios. These scenarios will consider (1) the scope and type of high-need, high-cost subpopulations served (2); the PACE model adaptations required; (3) competing programs and services; and (4) the impact of current and potential state and federal policy constraints.

Across the range of scenarios, the project developed both scale and spread strategies for achieving broader PACE 2.0 dissemination. In large population areas, the scale strategy sought to establish PACE 2.0 organizations that serve a high number of people. For smaller population areas, the spread strategy focused on establishing a larger number of PACE 2.0 organizations serving significantly more communities than currently served. A modified spread strategy that addresses rural areas was also included in the project aims. To propel PACE 2.0's growth under these strategies, the project communicated its findings and shared its resources with current or prospective providers, state and federal policy makers, and potential partners interested in contracting for PACE 2.0 services.

COVID-19 Pandemic Impact on PACE

Like all health care providers in the world, the COVID-19 pandemic had a monumental impact on the operations of PACE programs as well as the lives of PACE participants and staff. Unprecedented in scope and unpredictable in its behavior as a disease, this pandemic impacted the availability of center-based services as adult day care centers were forced to close for many months to help curb the spread of the virus. Similarly, face-to-face care was drastically restricted with most interactions with patients limited to "virtual" format, also known as "telehealth visits" (phone calls and Zoom sessions). Despite these limitations in access, the need for social services and support intensified, which forced all PACE providers to adapt their practices.

Throughout PACE operations, the pandemic pushed the model to be ever more creative and resilient in providing care to community-dwelling older adults. It was also necessary to support staff members who were often placed in care environments where personal safety was unknown. Through leadership at the local level and the national efforts of the National PACE Association, each PACE program continued to operate and maintain service lines. Although PACE programs did encounter COVID infections with the associated morbidity and mortality, programs consistently noted lower hospitalization rates during the pandemic and during prepandemic times. **For many reasons, there was a sense of national reckoning on the use of nursing homes for the care of large numbers of older adults in the United States. This has brought additional focus on the advantages and benefits of a comprehensive, community-based program like PACE.**

Summary

The Program of All-Inclusive Care for the Elderly (PACE) was started with humble beginnings in a Chinese American community in San Francisco. The idealism and sound design of that early model, along with continued refinement and adaptation to the political climate and available financing structures at the national and state levels, have enabled PACE to reach thousands of older adults and have allowed for sustained community residence within a cost-controlled (capitated) program design that depends heavily on the interdisciplinary team to provide person-centered, high-quality care.

Suggested Reading

1. Abt Associates, Inc. Evaluation of the program of all-inclusive care for the elderly (PACE) demonstration, 1998.
2. Eng E, Pedulla J, Eleazer GP, et al. Program of all-inclusive care for the elderly (PACE): an innovative model of integrated geriatric care and financing. J Am Geriatr Soc. 1997;45:223–32.
3. Ghosh A, Schmitz R, Brown R. Effects of PACE on costs, nursing home admissions, and mortality: 2006-2011. Mathematica Policy Research Report, 2014.
4. Gross DL, Temkin-Greener H, Kunitz S, et al. The growing pains of integrated health care for the elderly: lesson from the expansion of PACE. Millibank Q. 2004;82:257–82.

Chapter 4
Evaluating the Effectiveness of PACE

Sean Hennessy and Bruce Kinosian

Introduction

The Program of All-inclusive Care for the Elderly (PACE) is a care model for community-dwelling older adults who are at high risk for hospitalization and nursing home (NH) placement. PACE provides long-term support services (LTSS) that are integrated with multidisciplinary, capitated healthcare. PACE serves adults aged 55 and above who are eligible for nursing home care with the goal of improving the quality of life by enhancing people's ability to live in the community for as long as they desire. More than 98% of participants are enrolled in either both Medicaid and Medicare (dual eligible) or Medicaid alone (single cap). PACE serves a high-need population that has an average of 5.8 chronic conditions per enrollee; 46% of them have dementia, and 60% have limitations in at least three basic activities of daily living (ADLs) (e.g., dressing, bathing, transferring, toileting, eating, walking).

Despite the high level of need that characterizes the PACE population, more than 95% of PACE enrollees are community dwelling, and the rate of PACE disenrollment other than death is historically below 8 per 100 participants per year, but with a range among programs of 3–40/100 participants. Recently, a PACE-sponsored survey reported that 96.6% of family members were satisfied with the support provided by PACE and that 97.5% of family caregivers would recommend PACE to

S. Hennessy (✉)
Division of Epidemiology, Department of Biostatistics, Epidemiology and Informatics, University of Pennsylvania Perelman School of Medicine, Philadelphia, PA, USA
e-mail: hennessy@pennmedicine.upenn.edu

B. Kinosian
Department of Medicine, University of Pennsylvania Perelman School of Medicine, Philadelphia, PA, USA
e-mail: Bruce.Kinosian@pennmedicine.upenn.edu

M. K. McNabney (ed.), *Community-Based Integrated Care for Older Adults*,
https://doi.org/10.1007/978-3-031-05137-1_4

someone in a similar situation. Importantly, of the half of enrollees' family members who reported a high caregiver burden at the time of PACE enrollment, 58% reported that their burden was reduced after enrollment.

Despite these encouraging outcomes, policy makers, including federal and state legislators and program administrators, rely on comparative evidence about the effectiveness of PACE vs other models of care to inform decisions about the provision of government-funded LTSS and healthcare. In 2014, Gosh et al. of Mathematica Policy Research [1], under contract with the Assistant Secretary for Policy and Evaluation (ASPE) in the Department of Health and Human Services, critically evaluated comparative studies of PACE that were conducted from 1997 (the year that PACE was established as a permanent benefit of Medicaid and Medicare) to 2013. This chapter reviews and updates, with more recent studies, the evidence presented in Ghosh's 2014 ASPE review concerning PACE's effectiveness. Before reviewing this evidence, we first discuss issues related to research designs and comparator groups for evaluating the effectiveness of complex, longitudinal models, such as PACE.

Research Designs and Comparator Groups for Evaluating the Effectiveness of PACE

Randomized trials generally provide the highest level of evidence evaluating the effectiveness of medical interventions, such as drugs, devices, and surgical procedures. However, because of legal, ethical, and logistical considerations, randomized trials are infrequently used to measure the effectiveness of care models, such as PACE. As noted by Ghosh et al. [1], no randomized trials have examined the effectiveness of PACE, and such trials would probably be prohibited by law since PACE is an established benefit of Medicaid and Medicare, so it cannot be withheld from eligible persons. In the absence of randomized trials, policy makers must rely on evidence from nonrandomized designs, such as cohort studies. Cohort studies ideally enroll groups of people who, because of real-life circumstances, are new recipients of different treatments—in this case, models of care. Cohort studies then tabulate within-person changes in repeatable measures, such as quality of life, and/or rates of outcomes, such as death. These metrics are compared between treatment groups, often matching or otherwise adjusting for measured baseline imbalances between the groups. Failure to observe each subject from the point of entry into the care model risks introducing *prevalent cohort bias*, in which failure to capture early events results in distorted estimates of the effect being measured.

The primary weakness of nonrandomized cohort studies is the possibility that the groups being compared—in this case, people receiving care under different models—differ with respect to unmeasured baseline factors that affect the study outcome, a possibility known as *unmeasured confounding*. This is particularly true in models such as PACE, where enrollment is voluntary on the part of both the beneficiary and the PACE interdisciplinary team (usually if the IDT feels that the individual cannot be maintained safely in the community). This unmeasured confounding, driven in large part by unobserved selection factors, is the main reason why nonrandomized studies generally provide less compelling evidence of effectiveness than randomized trials do. Unmeasured confounding can play a larger a role in studies where the outcome is the *absolute level* of a binary variable (e.g., death) or a nonbinary variable (e.g., quality of life) than when the outcome is the *change* from preenrollment to postenrollment in a variable (e.g., the change in a person's quality of life). This is because examining within-person changes uses each person as her/his own control in addition to the control provided by the external comparator group.

In studying the effectiveness of the PACE model, it is important to consider whether all PACE programs are similar enough to warrant considering them equivalent. PACE programs differ with respect to many factors that might affect performance, such as the number of enrollees served, case mix, capitated payment level, staffing model, team composition, time that medical directors devote to medical practice, racial/ethnic similarity between enrollees and staff, the types of housing resources participants have (e.g., whether in private residences, group housing, or assisted living facilities), and the types of services provided. However, because PACE programs are all authorized under the same federal legislation and offer a relatively standard package of services, the studies that have compared PACE to external comparators usually have considered individual PACE programs to be equivalent, despite the four- to five-time variation found among PACE programs for a variety of process and clinical outcomes, including hospitalization, readmission, death in hospital, use of skilled nursing facilities (SNFs) for postacute care, and use of antipsychotic medications. The variation among PACE programs raises the challenge for evaluators as to whether a fair answer to the question of the effectiveness of PACE should reflect the model's highest performers, the median program, or all programs.

The choice of a comparator population has proven challenging for investigators as well, due in part to the voluntary nature of PACE participation, as well as the ability of PACE programs to support individuals in the community with resource needs far beyond traditional home and community-based service (HCBS) programs, who would otherwise enter nursing facilities for the long term. Perhaps the most commonly used external comparator group in the studies of PACE is recipients of home and community-based services (HCBSs) for the aged and disabled that are covered by Medicaid through waivers authorized by Section 1915 (c) of the Social Security Act (i.e., waivered HCBS). Like PACE, HCBS waiver programs provide in-home and other community-based services designed to support nursing-home-eligible Medicare-Medicaid dual enrollees to remain in community dwellings rather than enter long-term nursing facility care. Thus, HCBS programs are an intuitively appealing potential comparator group for the evaluation of PACE since one could imagine a hypothetical randomized trial that assigned nursing-home-eligible, dually enrolled persons seeking to remain in the community to either PACE or HCBS. Despite the intuitive appeal of this comparison, differences between PACE and HCBS waiver programs may affect the comparability of the groups that enroll in each program. For example, PACE but not most HCBS waiver programs provide multidisciplinary healthcare and closely integrated social support services at an adult day center. Because of such differences, the overall population served by HCBS waiver programs may have less medical comorbidity, cognitive impairment, and functional disability than that served by PACE. On the other hand, some HCBS recipients are homebound and therefore may be more functionally impaired than the average PACE participant, who is generally able to attend PACE day centers. There is probably a subset of the HCBS population—which itself is many times larger than the PACE population—that is comparable to the population of PACE enrollees. However, identifying such a subset is challenging at best and possibly unachievable for studies that rely exclusively on administrative healthcare data, which lack important prognostic information like ADL performance, cognitive impairment, housing, and strength of family support. In addition, because HCBS waiver programs probably vary more in their structure and provision of services than PACE programs do, comparisons between PACE and HCBS depend heavily on the nature of the services provided by the specific HCBS waiver programs being studied.

After HCBS waiver enrollees, the most commonly used external comparator group in PACE evaluations is new entrants to long-term nursing home care. However, persons receiving long-term nursing home care have higher overall levels of medical comorbidity, cognitive impairment, and functional disability than PACE enrollees and further may have less access to informal (i.e., unpaid) caregivers, which enables PACE enrollees to remain living in the community. Thus, new entrants to long-term nursing facility care probably do not constitute a valid comparator group for the evaluation of PACE, particularly for examining PACE's effectiveness in avoiding placement in a long-term nursing facility, although a portion of new entrants to nursing facilities are probably similar to more functionally impaired PACE participants.

Other external comparators in PACE evaluations have included people who had been offered PACE but declined and enrollees in managed LTSS (MLTSS) programs. Because of the differences between these populations and PACE enrollees, including autoenrollment in many MLTSS programs, these comparator groups are also challenging. The CMS Financial Alignment Initiative programs, which align an MLTSS program with dual-eligible special need plans (D-SNP), providing an integrated provision of Medicare and Medicaid HCBS benefits, might be comparable to PACE, although evaluations of those integrated programs have been challenging (https://innovation.cms.gov/innovation-models/financial-alignment).

Evaluation of the Effectiveness of PACE

The 2014 report produced by Ghosh et al. rated the level of evidence of effectiveness provided by each of the 22 studies that they identified. The authors *rated none as "strong"* (which they defined as a randomized controlled trial design), *four as "moderate-to-strong"* (nonrandomized design with a comparison group, regression adjustment, and established baseline equivalence on measured variables), *seven as* "*moderate*" (nonrandomized design with comparison group and regression adjustment but without established baseline equivalence on measured variables), *six as* "*moderate-to-weak*" (nonrandomized design with comparison group but without regression adjustment or baseline equivalence), and *five as* "*weak*" (comparison across PACE sites without a non-PACE comparison group). Below we summarize and update the discussion of studies evaluating the effectiveness of PACE in improving different outcomes of interest.

Effectiveness in Reducing Mortality

The 2014 review by Ghosh et al. identified two studies that it rated as providing moderate-to-strong evidence (although conducted in a single state), two studies rated as providing moderate evidence, and two studies rated as providing weak evidence about PACE's effectiveness in reducing mortality. In both studies rated as providing moderate-to-strong evidence, PACE enrollees had lower mortality than HCBS enrollees. The study by Wieland [2], following an inception cohort of new South Carolina LTSS users through HCBS, nursing homes, and PACE, found median survival in PACE (4.2 years) nearly double those entering a nursing home (2.3 years) and exceeding those entering HCBS (3.5 years), after adjusting for a 3-year mortality risk at entry.

In their subsequent study for ASPE, MPR [3] documented the results of a cohort study that examined new entrants to PACE across eight states from 2006 to 2008. Entrants to PACE in these states were compared to two different comparison groups: (1) matched Medicare beneficiaries who were *either* entrants to waivered HCBS programs or nursing home entrants with stays of 21 days or longer (to reduce the possibility that the stays identified in administrative claims were skilled nursing facility (SNF) stays rather than long-term nursing home stays) and (2) matched Medicare beneficiaries who were new entrants to waivered HCBS programs alone, i.e., excluding nursing home entrants. The rationale for using two comparator groups was the previously mentioned concerns that HCBS entrants may be, on average, less medically complex than PACE entrants and, conversely, that the group composed of waivered HCBS entrants and nursing home entrants may be, on average, more medically complex and frail than PACE entrants. Members of the comparison groups were matched with PACE entrants within a state on a multivariable score (i.e., propensity score), which included preenrollment demographics, chronic conditions, and health service utilization and costs. Matching was successful in balancing the study groups based on measured baseline factors, although propensity score matching is known to potentially increase unobserved differences that are inversely related to the observed matching measures. Deaths occurring in the first 6 months of enrollment were not counted since these were deemed unlikely to be affected by the choice of care model. Adjusted mortality rates from months 6 to 60 were lower in the PACE group than in both the HCBS + nursing home comparator group and the HCBS-alone comparator group. The investigators were cautious in interpreting the lower mortality in PACE entrants as an effect of PACE, citing the possibility that terminally ill patients or other unmeasured selection effects might have caused the difference.

A cohort study reported in a 2016 report for Massachusetts [4] used an inception cohort of LTSS participants, comparing PACE entrants in Massachusetts to Medicare-Medicaid dual enrollees in that state who were matched on both static and time-varying measures of disease burden and health service utilization. Rather than using propensity score methods, the investigators used direct matching on demographic measures, as well as a claim-based frailty index (the JEN frailty index (JFI)) and clinical trajectory, defined by the temporal pattern of utilization prior to enrollment. Subjects were followed for an average of 32 months. Mortality was 19% lower for PACE entrants in the first year of follow-up (hazard ratio 0.81; 95% confidence interval, 0.71–0.93) but similar overall (hazard ratio 1.03; 95% confidence interval, 0.95–1.11). The higher baseline utilization of nursing homes in the comparator group confirmed the hypothesis that PACE cares for a more complex group of beneficiaries than HCBS waiver programs, diverting some from directly entering nursing homes, and supporting a mixed HCBS/nursing home population for comparison to PACE.

Thus, there is some suggestion from existing studies that PACE may reduce mortality. However, given the likelihood that the PACE participants and the comparator groups in these studies differed with respect to unmeasured confounding factors and considering the impossibility of comparing within-person preenrollment vs postenrollment changes in the death rate—as we might for repeatable measures like quality of life—we cannot reasonably conclude that PACE is effective in reducing mortality. Further, while mortality may be a very salient outcome for comparing healthcare models for many patient populations, longer life is not necessarily the most desirable outcome for all PACE participants. This is because the main goal of PACE is to improve the quality of life by enhancing people's ability to live in the community for as long as they desire. Achieving this goal could reasonably result in reduced, increased, or no change in mortality, depending on the circumstances and preferences of the individual PACE participant, many of whom are impaired, frail, and experiencing significant morbidity. Thus, even if we could measure with certainty PACE's effect on mortality, doing so would not necessarily provide the most salient measure for assessing PACE's effectiveness. As illustrated by the JEN Massachusetts PACE study, delay in nursing home entry in a cohort at high risk of death can reduce early mortality yet has little effect on longer-term mortality, while increasing the time individuals remain at home. Home time, measured in a variety of ways, is increasingly becoming a summative measure of overall HCBS program quality and effectiveness [5].

Effectiveness in Reducing Hospitalization

The 2014 review by Ghosh et al. identified two studies that it rated as providing moderate-to-strong evidence, three providing moderate evidence, and five providing weak or moderate-to-weak evidence about the effectiveness of PACE in reducing hospitalization. The comparator groups used in these studies included HCBS enrollees, nursing home residents, people who had been offered PACE but declined, enrollees in Medicaid-only managed long-term care, and other groups. The report's authors concluded that the strongest studies found that PACE enrollees have fewer inpatient hospitalizations than comparators and that there was some evidence that more mature PACE sites have lower hospitalization rates than newer sites.

Segelman et al. [6] performed a study funded by the National PACE Association that examined the effect of PACE on inpatient hospitalization. However, this study did not include a comparator group for which the investigators had individual-level data, instead using hospitalization benchmarks for dual-eligible HCBS participants. While not restricted to new entrants (and so subject to prevalent cohort bias from either a healthy survivor effect among PACE participants or adverse selection among incident HCBS participants), PACE hospitalizations over 3 years (2008–2010) were 40% less than the dual HCBS benchmark (539 hospitalizations/1000 beneficiaries vs 962 hospitalizations/1000 beneficiaries) and less than half for potentially avoidable hospitalizations (PAH) (100 PAH/1000 beneficiaries vs 252 PAH/1000 beneficiaries). Subsequent studies by the National PACE Association covering 2014–2016 and 2017–2019 have found similar rates of hospitalization (504–590/1000). Importantly, Segelman documented a five-time variation in hospitalizations among PACE programs, highlighting the question of whether model effectiveness should be judged by the best programs, the median program, or all the programs of a model. (This is analogous to whether the efficacy of a transcatheter aortic valve replacement (TAVR) should be judged by the outcomes of the most proficient surgeons, the median surgeon, or all surgeons performing the procedure.)

Thus, available studies provide consistent evidence suggesting that PACE reduces the frequency of hospital admission, which is a reasonable goal for a program seeking to keep participants living in the community. However, given the potential for unmeasured confounding and the studies' inability to compare individual-level pre- vs postenrollment changes in a repeated measure, this suggestion of benefit is far from definitive. On balance, measures typically used to guard against withholding needed care (mortality), On balance, the weight of studies suggests positive PACE effects.

Effectiveness in Reducing Nursing Facility Admission/Utilization

The 2014 review by Ghosh et al. identified one study rated as providing moderate-to-strong evidence, one as providing moderate evidence, and four as providing moderate-to-weak or weak evidence regarding the effectiveness of PACE in reducing nursing facility utilization, a stated goal of PACE. These studies used a variety of comparator groups, including HCBS enrollees, people who had been offered PACE but declined, enrollees in Medicaid-only managed long-term care, and other groups. The review concluded that the strongest evidence suggested that PACE participants have higher rates of nursing facility admission than comparators. However, none of the studies distinguished between skilled nursing facility (SNF) and long-term nursing facility stays, which limits their interpretability as one of the approaches used by PACE programs to reduce hospitalizations is to substitute subacute care in nursing facilities. A clearer specification of the question of PACE's impact on nursing facility admission would focus on long-term institutionalization (currently thought of as more than 100 days in a facility).

The eight-state ASPE study reported in 2015 by Ghosh et al., which was discussed above, also examined nursing facility utilization. The study compared PACE entrants to entrants of HCBS programs, who were matched to PACE entrants in the same state based on a multivariable score. The results suggested that while PACE participants were more likely to receive care at an SNF or long-term nursing facility, they were less likely to have stays of 90 days or longer in any given interval. However, cumulative rates of long-term nursing home stay were similar between groups, suggesting that PACE may delay, but not prevent, long-term nursing home stays. The authors hypothesized that PACE may use short-term nursing home stays to avoid or shorten some hospitalizations, confirming the reported practice of PACE programs.

The 2016 Massachusetts PACE study by JEN Associates evaluated the number of full or partial months of nursing facility residency during 6.5 years of follow-up. PACE entrants had a 28% lower number of nursing facility months than the comparator group of Medicare-Medicaid dual enrollees, with both having a lower average number of nursing facility months among beneficiaries (4.5 vs 6.3) and also a lower number of nursing facility months among those beneficiaries residing in nursing facilities (13.3 vs 21.2). Due to the careful direct matching on clinical trajectory as well as frailty, a strong and clear 20-month delay in nursing facility entry is seen (Fig. 4.1). This contrasts with the nursing facility entry reported by Ghosh [3] for Massachusetts (one of the eight studied states), which had a different comparator group (propensity-matched HCBS without any matching on the clinical trajectory of frailty). While the PACE rate exceeds the HCBS rate in the later months (36+), that rate applies to a population that by 36 months is 60% of the population at the study index. The delay in early NH entry, paired with the mortality in the high-risk population, leads to the lower overall months of long-term institutionalization.

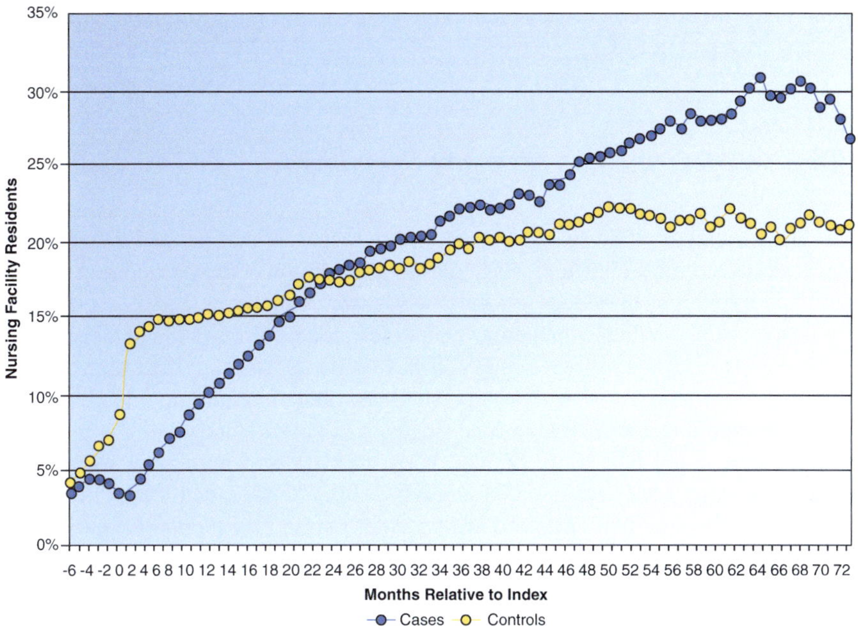

Fig. 4.1 Nursing facility residency in months from the JEN PACE Study Index

As the JEN authors concluded:

> PACE in Massachusetts met its goal of maintaining enrollees in a community care setting—at least through the first 20 months after enrollment. Nursing facility residency increased rapidly in the controls after the index date but climbed more slowly among the PACE enrollees. In both groups, residency in nursing grew slowly between months 21 and 41, increasing from 17–18% to 21–23%. The sustained PACE effect over the observation period is statistically significantly, representing a PACE population reduction of 28% in any residency months and a reduction of 38% in total NF residency months per patient.

A cohort study published in 2017 by Segelman et al. [7] compared new entrants to PACE and waivered HCBS in 12 states. Adjusting for baseline variables, they found that PACE entrants were 31% less likely than HCBS entrants to enter long-term nursing home care. In addition, among those who entered long-term nursing home care, PACE entrants were more functionally and cognitively impaired than HCBS entrants, again consistent with delay in NH entry, suggesting that PACE enabled participants to remain living in the community longer at lower levels of functional and cognitive performance than did HCBS programs.

Thus, existing studies provide some evidence that PACE is effective in delaying or avoiding the long-term use of nursing facilities; PACE also uses short nursing facility stays instead of for more costly hospital admissions or to provide respite to informal caregivers. The low (less than 5%) point prevalence of nursing home utilization in this population certified as eligible for nursing home care itself suggests that PACE is effective in supporting its participants to remain living in the community, where a comparable community rate of NH entry might be three times the rate observed in PACE.

Effect on Medicaid and Medicare Spending

The 2014 review by Ghosh et al. identified two studies that it rated as providing moderate-to-strong evidence, three studies as providing moderate evidence, and one study as providing moderate-to-weak evidence concerning PACE's effect on Medicare and/or Medicaid spending. The review concluded that the evidence from the strongest studies suggests that PACE has no demonstrable effect on Medicare spending but is associated with higher Medicaid spending, although the excess in Medicaid spending declined with time since a participant's entry into the program. Their review noted one study [8] that used sophisticated regression methods to decompose costs of HCBS and NH entrants across 80 demographic, clinical, and frailty measures and then projected an expected cost for PACE entrants, to be compared to their actual Medicaid expenditures, finding the state Medicaid PACE rate 28% below the expected cost for those same participants. While the authors felt the study had only moderate strength because it did not establish baseline equivalence, the study design dealt with the seemingly intractable issues of selection bias by using the PACE participants as their own controls based on their characteristics and the relationship of those characteristics to expected costs. The review also noted that because of changes to Medicare capitation formulas, which have been implemented since the completion of the studies, and the variation in state Medicaid rate methodologies, the findings on Medicare and Medicaid spending may be limited by time and place. For example, the Wieland study covered the years 1997–2006, with substantial changes in Medicaid rate setting in the interim.

The eight-state ASPE study by Ghosh et al. [3] also examined Medicaid and Medicare spending in PACE entrants compared to (1) HCBS entrants and nursing home entrants and (2) waivered HCBS enrollees alone. That study found little or no association between the enrollment care model and Medicare spending but found an association with higher Medicaid spending in PACE, especially compared to the HCBS-alone comparator group. These results varied somewhat by state, which was expected since Medicaid capitation formulas vary by state.

Thus, available evidence suggests that, using capitation formulas that were current as of the time that the studies were conducted, PACE is cost-neutral to Medicare but in the short term may result in higher Medicaid spending than alternative models of care, potentially driven by the lower mortality the same study found. As with the evaluation of the effect of PACE on other outcomes, the lack of an ideal comparator group for PACE enrollees precludes definitive conclusions about whether these findings represent true effects. The approach taken by Wieland [8], cited in Ghosh, where the costs are modeled among the potential comparator population and then applied to the PACE population may correct for the confounding effects of both mortality and unobserved selection factors. Given that per-enrollee taxpayer costs for PACE and other managed LTSS programs are formulaic, their predictability is a desirable feature for program administrators.

An alternative view on the higher Medicaid spending can be based on the JEN Massachusetts study, focusing only on the trade-off of NH use and Medicaid spending in Massachusetts. Using the JEN study rates of NH use, and months of observations, paired with Massachusetts' PACE, HCBS, and NH rates from the Ghosh 2015 ASPE study, the PACE cohort would have received $358 million in capitated payments over 7 years of the study for the 3456 PACE participants, or $103,000 per participant ($3197 per beneficiary per month (*pbpm*)). For the 3456 LTSS comparison cohort members, the cost would have been $326 million, or $94,000 per participant ($2817 pbpm). Given the common preference of individuals to remain at home and not live in long-term institutional settings, the 38% reduction in nursing facility residency months is likely well worth the difference of $380 pbpm. The recent experience in 2020 of the pandemic risks of congregate living arrangements, such as nursing facilities, would likely increase the value of living in the community.

Effectiveness in Improving Potential Metrics of Quality of Care

The 2014 review by Ghosh et al. found one study rated as providing moderate-to-strong evidence, one as providing moderate-to-weak evidence, and four as providing weak evidence regarding the effects of PACE vs other care models on potential metrics of quality of care. The study rated as providing moderate-to-strong evidence was conducted by Beauchamp et al. and identified new enrollees of PACE and new enrollees of HCBS programs in eight states and communicated its results in a non-peer-reviewed report. Subjects were first interviewed 18 months to 5 years after program enrollment and again a year later. The study found that at the first interview, PACE participants were more likely to have a living will and an advance directive and less likely to experience pain that interfered with normal routine than did waivered HCBS enrollees. However, because subjects had been enrolled in the respective programs for at least 18 months before the first interview, it is unclear how much of the observed difference was present at baseline, how much was an effect of PACE, and how much of the results were affected by a nonrandom loss to follow-up. PACE enrollees were much more likely than HCBS enrollees to report receiving preventive care in the past year, such as influenza vaccination and vision and hearing screening, which because of the time period assessed seems more likely to have been affected by PACE than an ever-before measure, such as having an advance directive. Thus, this single study provides some evidence that PACE provides better preventive care than do waivered HCBS programs.

The 2014 review by Ghosh et al. also described two related studies that examined, among new PACE participants, the association between PACE program characteristics and ADL limitations and the frequency of urinary incontinence measured at 12 months after PACE enrollment and adjusting for baseline values of these variables. The investigators found that measured PACE characteristics, including the self-rated performance of the PACE care team, having a full-time medical director, having a trained geriatrician as a medical director, and an ethnic mix of PACE nonprofessional staff that more closely matched that of the participants, were all associated with fewer limitations in performing basic ADLs and less frequent urinary incontinence. Thus, while these two related studies provide evidence suggesting that the characteristics of PACE programs can influence ADL limitations and the frequency of urinary incontinence, it does not provide any basis for comparing the performance of PACE with other models of care.

Effectiveness as Measured by Satisfaction with Care and Quality of Life

The 2014 review by Ghosh et al. identified one study providing moderate-to-strong evidence, one providing moderate evidence, and one providing moderate-to-weak evidence about the effectiveness of PACE when it comes to satisfaction with care and quality of life. The study rated as providing moderate-to-strong evidence was the above-described study by Beauchamp et al., which identified new enrollees of PACE and new enrollees of HCBS programs in eight states. Investigators surveyed respondents about their overall satisfaction with the quality of care they received from PACE or HCBS, satisfaction with their medical care, and satisfaction with personal assistance. Both PACE and HCBS enrollees reported very high levels of satisfaction with the care they received. Of the few observed differences in satisfaction and quality of care measures, some favored PACE and some favored waivered HCBS.

The study that was rated as providing moderate evidence surveyed PACE participants and a comparison group of individuals who expressed interest in PACE and received a home visit in preparation for enrollment but who did not enroll in PACE. Limitations of the study include the potential noncomparability of PACE enrollees and PACE decliners and the survey response rate of 44%. Thus, although this study ascertained information about the quality of life, satisfaction with care, caregiver burden, and other important metrics, limitations of the study design preclude us from giving the results much evidentiary weight.

Thus, descriptive survey data suggest that PACE participants and their family members are satisfied with healthcare and other services provided by PACE. For example, survey data reported by PACE suggest that 96.6% of family members are satisfied with the support provided by PACE and that 97.5% of family caregivers would recommend PACE to someone in a similar situation. The low disenrollment rate from PACE suggests a high level of satisfaction with the model and with participation in the model throughout the first year, lowering the voluntary disenrollment rate to less than half of the overall 8% rate.

A current summative quality measure, to be used by the Centers for Medicare & Medicaid Services (CMS) in their Direct Contracting and Primary Care First demonstrations, is to use home time—capturing the time that individuals are alive and residing in the community. While there have been no studies of PACE that directly measure home time, the delay in long-term nursing facility admission, coupled with the reduction in hospitalization, likely suggests a strong PACE effect on improving home time.

An area where home time has been recently used is in hospice care, where it is a measure of the lack of institutional use (hospitals and nursing facilities) in the last 6 months of life [9]. While there is not a comparable PACE study of home time, recent analyses by the National PACE Association have found over 45% of PACE participants having no hospital use in the year of their death, with less than 20% dying in hospitals (compared to 34% among all community-dwelling dual-eligible Medicare beneficiaries aged 75 or more), again suggesting that PACE should perform well on the newer "days at home" measures.

Summary

Available data suggest that, compared to external comparison groups, PACE is associated with reduced mortality, reduced time in hospital, a delay in long-term nursing home residence and a reduced long-term use of nursing facilities, an increase in short-term use of nursing facilities as a substitute for hospital use, and is cost-neutral to Medicare. PACE may increase costs to Medicaid through an individual's lifetime, but at a cost well worth the delay in nursing home residence. However, the lack of evidence from randomized trials, and the challenges inherent in conducting and interpreting nonrandomized comparisons of care models, such as the potential lack of comparability of reference groups, preclude us from drawing firm conclusions about the effectiveness of PACE in affecting these outcome measures. Nevertheless, there is reasonable evidence that compared to new LTSS beneficiaries choosing either HCBS or nursing facility use—probably the most appropriate comparator—PACE improves the metrics of desired preventive care, such as influenza vaccination and hearing and vision screening. Additional pieces of evidence for the success of PACE are the low prevalence of nursing facility residence in this population certified as eligible for nursing facility care, the low rate of disenrollment from PACE, and the high level of satisfaction with the care received, as reported by the PACE participants and their family members. These comparisons come from the "whole of PACE" evaluations (either nationally or within a state or group of states), thus ignoring the variation among PACE programs in each of these measures and incorporating the performance of lower-performing programs in judging the effectiveness of the care model. A focus on the median program or the set of higher-performing programs might be a better reflection of the value of the PACE care model.

The rapid expansion of for-profit PACE programs since their inclusion in 2016 [10] raises other cautions about using a "whole of PACE" focus, even though the model has been remarkably robust to those evaluations, despite a five-time variation in performance across multiple measures.

In the past two decades since PACE obtained a permanent provider status, there has been a proliferation of care models seeking to replicate the key elements of PACE, with a focus on integrating Medicare-funded management of complex medical needs and Medicaid-funded services and support of functional disabilities, with the even more recent recognition of the importance of housing to successful integration. The complexities of studying similar high-need populations have created similar challenges for CMS [11]. An approach that uses predictive modeling for costs, utilization, and summative measures such as "home time" to establish expected outcomes to compare to a program's observed performance, combined with assessments of outcomes that matter to patients and their families (e.g. pain, physical function, attainment of patient care goals, caregiver burden, stress, and workforce participation of family caregivers), may provide evidence of effects across different care models that can be used to assess comparative effectiveness. When constructed at the program level, such measures should allow a comparison of models for their median practitioner, rather than assume that all examples of a care model have equal fidelity and effectiveness. As more states move toward managed LTSS, the best comparator for care models will shift from traditional fee for service. This shift will necessitate benchmarking methods that account for the strong selection effects that drive participation in particular care models.

Despite the proliferation of alternatives, over three decades as a demonstration and then as a Medicare provider, PACE has become not only a benchmark for high-quality care, allowing some of Medicare's frailest beneficiaries to thrive in their communities, but also a challenging tale of the limits of health service research methods for documenting those effects.

References

1. Ghosh A, Orfield C, Schmitz R. Evaluating PACE: a review of the literature. Washington, DC: US Department of Health and Human Services; 2014.
2. Wieland D, Boland R, Baskins J, Kinosian B. Five-year survival in a program of all-inclusive care for elderly compared with alternative institutional and home-and community-based care. J Gerontol A Biol Sci Med Sci. 2010;65(7):721–6.
3. Ghosh A, Schmitz R, Brown R. Effect of PACE on cost, nursing home admission, and mortality: 2006-2010. Mathematica Policy Research; 2015.
4. JEN Associates, Inc. Massachusetts PACE evaluation: nursing facility residency and mortality—Summary Report. 2016.
5. Van Houtven CV, Smith VA, Sperber NR, Coffman CJ, Hastings SN. Advancing the science of population-based measures of home-time. Healthcare. 2020;8(4):100463. https://doi.org/10.1016/j.hjdsi.2020.100463.

6. Segelman M, Szydlowski J, Kinosian B, McNabney M, Raziano DB, Eng C, van Reenen C, Temkin-Greener H. Hospitalizations in the program of all-inclusive care for the elderly. J Am Geriatr Soc. 2014;62(2):320–4. https://doi.org/10.1111/jgs.12637.
7. Segelman M, Cai X, Van Reenen C, Temkin-Greener H. Transitioning from community-based to institutional long-term care: comparing 1915 (c) waiver and PACE enrollees. The Gerontologist. 2017;57(2):300–8.
8. Wieland D, Kinosian B, Stallard E, Boland R. Does Medicaid pay more to a program of all-inclusive care for the elderly (PACE) than for fee-for-service long-term care?. J Gerontol A Biol Sci Med Sci. 2013;68(1):47–55.
9. Groff AC, Colla CH. TH Lee "days spent at home—a patient-centered goal and outcome". N Engl J Med. 2016;375(17):1610–2.
10. Gonzalez L. A focus on the program of all-inclusive care for the elderly (PACE). J Aging Soc Policy. 2017;29(5):475–90. https://doi.org/10.1080/08959420.2017.1281092.
11. Ornstein K, Levine DM, Leff B. The underappreciated success of home-based primary care: next steps for CMS' independence at home. J Am Geriatr Soc. 2021;2021:1–4. https://doi.org/10.1111/jgs.17426.

Part III
The Organization and Management of PACE

Chapter 5
Leadership in PACE

Ellen Garcia

This chapter is intended to describe the keys to success in PACE leadership, which have worked effectively for the author. Each PACE program is so unique. These ideas are offered from a place of humility, recognizing that for each PACE leader, the journey continues to unfold with each new challenge faced.

Throughout this chapter, the experience of one PACE site (Providence ElderPlace) will be shared as examples to highlight the key points. The length and intensity of time spent guiding a PACE program will influence perspective and insight. Over 20 years of leadership within PACE by the author serves as the reference point for content and recommendations made in this chapter.

PACE leaders assume their positions from a wide range of experience, including acute care and hospice leadership, and many will have limited knowledge of what leading a PACE program truly means. There can be a steep learning curve, which can be daunting. All established PACE leaders can recall the transition to the world of PACE. Preparing to assume a PACE leadership role will typically begin with reaching out to mentors and colleagues from across the country. In response to requests for guidance, one will need to identify a PACE community of passionate leaders who can answer inquiries with enthusiasm and candor. With its innovative approach to care and its deep commitment to serving frail older adults through the end of their lives, PACE offers an opportunity for creative leadership in care delivery systems and health policy advocacy.

This chapter has been organized into the following focus areas:

- The Call to Serve—Creating a Sense of Mission.
- Begin with a Leadership Team.
- A Vision for Growth.

E. Garcia (✉)
Providence ElderPlace Oregon, Portland, OR, USA
e-mail: ellen.garcia@providence.org

M. K. McNabney (ed.), *Community-Based Integrated Care for Older Adults*,
https://doi.org/10.1007/978-3-031-05137-1_5

- Promoting "Value-Based Care" as a PACE Leader.
- The Devil Is in the Details.
- Integration of Palliative Care.
- Garnering Resources.

The Call to Serve—Creating a Sense of Mission

Much has been said about the critical importance of mission and vision in organizational leadership. In the context of PACE, which was conceived by a dedicated group of visionary leaders in San Francisco in the 1970s, first and foremost**, a leader must firmly embrace its integrated model of care**. It has been argued that PACE is the "Gold Standard" of care for frail older adults with complex medical and functional needs. By creating a capitated, comprehensive model that aligned incentives across the entire continuum of care, PACE offered a new solution outside of the walls of a nursing home. To effectively lead a PACE program, it is essential to be imbued with a sense of mission firmly rooted in the belief that this model offers the best care possible for this at-risk population. PACE is evidence based and is known to provide a high quality of care. **The ability to articulate a mission that centers on the desire to achieve quality outcomes is the first fundamental building block in PACE leadership**. This foundational connection to the dignity of PACE participants establishes the vision for the future in which excellent interdisciplinary work is sustained and thrives. It demands a steadfast dedication and the personal grit to weather whatever new challenge is presented. Serving in an organization primarily serving dual-eligible (Medicare/Medicaid) individuals, a PACE leader is often called upon to advocate for the poorest and most vulnerable. This advocacy is frequently toward audiences with a limited understanding of the complexity of serving older adults with multiple medical needs and limited natural social support. Advocacy is most successful when it is grounded in a sincere commitment to the PACE model and a mission of service. An authentic embrace of the core values underpins work and will shape success in this arena.

If the PACE program is part of a larger health system, the agency's mission may be defined externally from the PACE program. The very fact that a PACE program exists as part of the delivery system reflects a commitment from the sponsoring health care organization that PACE offers services consistent with their overarching mission. Many PACE programs are sponsored by faith-based health systems that have integrated mission leadership formation training into the fabric of their work. Independent successful PACE programs not affiliated with a sponsor also take time to articulate a mission as a guiding principle for their teams and strategies. This commitment to the mission of the PACE model of care becomes a touchstone to return to when faced with countless challenging decisions. In Providence ElderPlace, over 90% of respondents of annual employee engagement surveys report strong agreement with statements measuring the employee's "resonance with the mission."

Creating an organizational culture rooted in mission fosters a sense of meaning for team members, which contributes to higher employee satisfaction and longevity. Every day, when an interdisciplinary team confronts a complex set of needs and competing imperatives, the mission must remain its guiding principle in clinical decision-making. Effective leadership includes the cultivation of a lived mission that everyone on the team shares.

Begin with a Leadership Team

The founding leaders of PACE took painstaking efforts to codify the elements of a PACE program into the PACE protocols and ultimately the CMS PACE regulations. In their wisdom, it was recognized that an essential element for the success of the program was in defining key roles and qualifications for those providing direct service to participants. A leader within PACE very quickly realizes that it is going to take individuals with many areas of expertise to lead a PACE program. The creation of a leadership team should include key leaders in clinical care, operations, quality, finance, marketing, health plan, human resources, information technology, and strategy. It is recommended that this team also include leaders with discipline-specific backgrounds in social work, nursing, business, rehab, long-term care, and medicine. Surrounding leadership with talent will lead to shared leadership and stronger decisions. Creating an environment that fosters open communication and involvement by this broad base of talent leads to success.

Another essential skill of the leader is the ability to cultivate talent. **By focusing on creating an organization dedicated to ongoing learning and development of teams, the effectiveness of the leadership team strengthens as the PACE organization grows**. Whether a part of a larger health system or not, providing opportunities for leadership growth at every level of the PACE organization paves the way for ongoing success. Attendance at nationally sponsored education forums and participation in PACE-specific work groups offer natural opportunities to develop a "deep bench" of leaders within the PACE program.

One of the most important decisions a PACE leader makes is in the recruitment and retention of a strong medical director. Backgrounds vary and their leadership styles even more so. PACE leadership cannot underestimate the importance of the medical director's role. Together, you will be advocating for your PACE program and contributing to its success on both a clinical and financial basis. Medical directors may possess a range of skills and qualifications, from geriatrics to hospice/palliative care to family practice and pulmonary medicine to psychiatry. It is not the board certification, or the added MBA, that portends success. The real key is a steadfast dedication to the model, a willingness to champion it, and the ability to work within an interdisciplinary team. A medical director ultimately has accountability for the quality of care delivered in the PACE program. This is delineated in the PACE regulation. Equally important is critical leadership in utilization management and in building relationships with the medical community. PACE looks to medical directors to be educators for primary care providers, colleagues, interdisciplinary teams, and the community. A strong medical director becomes an effective spokesperson for PACE in government advocacy and frequently has a state and national profile. Their knowledge is invaluable in key operational decisions, such as the selection of an electronic health record or the implementation of care pathways. They also serve a critical role as a clinical consultant for challenging cases that frequently call into question ethical issues. With the medical complexity of those served, a strong PACE program needs a dedicated, clinically strong medical director who is also a strong leader. In larger programs, the scope of the work may require additional associate medical directors as well.

In 2020–2021, the world was confronting a pandemic that is unprecedented, with a disproportionate impact on frail older adults, especially those in congregate settings. This tested PACE leadership, and medical directors were instrumental in crafting effective responses through direct participation in command centers, research, and multifaceted infection prevention efforts. They also provided essential education to ensure safety for both participants and staff in the face of this threat.

Like all successful leaders, many will read numerous books addressing the various dimensions of their work. Leaders learn from the insights of others who have focused on establishing goals, holding teams accountable, and setting strategy that withstands the test of time. When considering the role of a PACE leader surrounded by dynamic leaders and clinicians, one should reflect on the human elements of leadership. This is captured eloquently by Margaret Wheatley, in her recent book Who Do We Choose to Be? Facing Reality, Claiming Leadership, Restoring Sanity. She posed the question, "'What is good leadership?' People in all places, of all ages, come up with the same descriptors. I feel confident that there is only one style, type, form of leadership that people respond well to. And they respond because it honors and supports them to be fully human." [1]

As PACE programs cultivate a dynamic PACE leadership team, including medical directors, it is important to consider the human elements of this work. By honoring the gifts that each individual colleague brings to the team, one strengthens collective leadership results and nurtures connections that respond to new opportunities.

A Vision for Growth

Two predictable drivers of success for a PACE program are census and utilization. This seems like such a simple, clear statement, but it is a central tenet of PACE leadership. What can program leadership do to instill an understanding of the critical intersection of these two driving factors? Ultimately, PACE is a health plan. Census (the number of beneficiaries served by the program) spreads the financial risk across many individuals. Recognizing that all PACE participants have high needs, a single outlier claim has the potential to impact the financial viability of a

PACE program. While PACE can focus on growth for the right reason of increasing access to the "gold standard" of care to more people, census also contributes to the long-term financial stability of the program. Many leaders who believe in the significant merits of PACE programs are shocked by the data that indicate that only one in ten persons eligible for PACE are currently being served [2].

For the past several years, the PACE program in Portland, OR, has incorporated growth as a strategic initiative. There was planning that resulted in expanded service areas, counties, and additional sites. This strategy builds the capacity to serve. There have been partnerships with other organizations providing adult day health services and co-located in housing. With the capital intensity and long lead times to develop PACE Centers, it will be necessary to creatively deploy clinical resources to meet a growing census. Several years ago, the term "PACE at Home" was coined to more effectively serve end-of-life participants and those with advanced dementia for whom center attendance becomes a negative experience. As the population served continues to evolve, the program is exploring many ways to broaden care in the community. Among PACE leaders, there is a recognition that many "baby boomers," a growing segment of those served, have no desire to participate in the group socialization experience that the PACE Center offers. In order to continue to grow the program, constant focus on the participant experience is vital. Sometimes, this requires great versatility.

For example, when confronted with the COVID-19 pandemic, PACE programs quickly pivoted from center-based adult day health activities to new forms of service delivery, such as telehealth. In response to mental health and the need for socialization, teams created innovative ways to continue to offer services and activities. This flexibility in program design is a component of census development.

Census growth strategies are addressed in other areas of this text and in the recent article by Gong & Fitzgerald [3]. Program leadership assumes a key role in placing census at the center of the PACE program. Mature PACE programs have established tools to increase the visibility of census at all levels within the organization. This is accomplished by sharing weekly dashboards that capture data on current enrollments, deaths, disenrollments, potential enrollments, and projected census. A simple Excel table is sufficient for this task; more sophisticated tools emerge over time. To increase efficiency, intake staff can be embedded at PACE sites while having their work supported by a central team of information referral specialists who take the initial referral call. By implementing a computerized customer referral database, leadership will be able to track, analyze, and trend the life cycle of a referral from the first inquiry call to enrollment. These detailed data are used constantly. On a monthly basis, referral and enrollment data can be reviewed with a special emphasis on the conversion rates of inquiries to enrollments. For example, Providence ElderPlace had a 45% conversion rate from eligible referral to enrollment in 2019. Through a careful analysis of the census referral management database, referral sources that result in the most likely enrollments can be targeted.

It is important to seek new opportunities to reach underserved communities of PACE-eligible participants. Outreach specialists are engaged in the day-to-day tasks of cultivating strong relationships with referral sources. Still, it is essential for executive leaders to leverage their positions to create connections and build trust for future referral development. This cultivates the importance of community partners and engages everyone in the organization with the challenge of census development. **PACE leadership may also be called upon to address tension that may arise between intake teams and interdisciplinary teams**. Recognizing that this tension can exist, leaders should speak clearly and openly about it while emphasizing that census growth is everyone's responsibility. This is important, nuanced work.

Historically, PACE programs were built on a budgeting model that was premised on staffing to achieve defined ratios of clinicians to the number of participants served. The realities of current financial performance may preclude adding additional staffing in anticipation of census growth. Certainly, when creating a new PACE Center, there must be staffing ahead of enrollments—this expense is built into the "pro-forma" at start-up. Existing PACE programs may need to utilize flexible staffing patterns to bridge the gap until they are able to justify the addition of interdisciplinary members or support staff. A frequent strategy is to hire individuals at a partial FTE (full-time equivalent), which can be increased as census grows. Over time, programs can augment discipline capacity with "extender" roles, such as physical therapy assistants, certified occupational therapy assistants, social work associates, and licensed practical nurses (LPNs). Existing PACE Center managers can serve in interim capacities when developing new sites. This has the added benefit of bringing an experienced leader to a new center to train to newly hired team members in the systems and structures of the organization.

Though census growth is foundational to the success of PACE programs, there are states that have placed "caps" on the number of PACE participants allowed for each PACE program in the state. This is a frequent strategy when the states themselves are facing budget shortfalls. Some programs have endured when the state redefined eligibility and many enrollees no longer qualified. Leaders must advocate for the removal of and/or the increase of caps. In the absence of success in state lobbying around census caps, this role shifts then to operational efficiency to sustain the PACE organization within a limited census.

Promoting "Value Based Care" as a PACE Leader

"PACE is identified as a model of care that fosters effectiveness in health and well-being, care utilization and costs," according to the National Academy of Medicine report "Effective Care for High-Need Patients" – Opportunities for Improving Outcomes, Value and Health [4]. When the Institute for Healthcare Improvement (IHI) coined the term "Triple Aim" as a framework for healthcare innovation in 2007, it highlighted the intersection of patient experience, population health outcomes, and costs. It was quickly recognized that the PACE model had been engaged in this type of value-based care delivery for years. As more and more mainstream health care dialogue is centered around population management, PACE is recognized for its skill in offering value-based care to a complex, high-need population.

Being able to articulate the place for PACE in driving solutions to address the rising cost of health care through population management has been a critical aspect of PACE leadership. A central dimension of PACE is knowing the participants very well and bringing the "voice of the participant" into our program operations and strategies. Within PACE, a tremendous amount of attention is focused on reducing the cost of care through efficiency and by delivering medically appropriate care. **There is an adage in PACE that the goal is to deliver "the Right care at the Right time in the Right place."** This continues to be an important, relevant leadership strategy. In the current health care climate, showcasing the role of PACE as value-based care is key to future considerations of an expanded role of the model. With the proliferation of Medicare Advantage plans and other dual-eligible products, PACE needs to continue to articulate its strength in serving a cohort that historically accounts for the highest spend for a health plan. Further, PACE enrollment results in outcomes that are significant for health plans: enrollee satisfaction, quality outcomes, and decreased utilization.

Some PACE programs embark on expense reduction efforts euphemistically called "Operational Improvement Plans." There is certainly a compelling case that health care costs are unstainable at the current trajectory. Costs for the highly skilled team that are needed in PACE require a constant review of expenses and the identification of opportunities to reduce. For example, PACE's commitment to the integration of highly skilled personnel in disciplines that are not required from a PACE regulatory perspective but contribute significantly to enhanced clinical care compels PACE to heighten the commitment to an efficient utilization of other resources. Some PACE programs have imbedded clinical pharmacists with geriatric expertise as well as mental health nurse practitioners. Neither of these disciplines is mentioned as a part of the "required IDT members" by the Centers for Medicare & Medicaid Services (CMS). However, serving complex geriatric participants has led some PACE programs to conclude that having these services integrated into the care delivery system will extend the capacity of the IDT to manage complex and larger panels of participants. Clinical pharmacists, speech therapists, behavioral health specialists, wound experts, and chaplains are examples of professionals who bring a wealth of expertise to the care delivery model. As programs grow, PACE leaders will rise to the challenge of integrating other important disciplines to create enhanced person-centered outcomes. The integration of behavioral health is also a leadership imperative as part of the effort to enroll "younger" more complex participants.

The Devil Is in the Details

The task of a PACE leader is to create an organizational culture that promotes consistent compliance with regulatory requirements and quality. **Executive leaders need to be very conversant in PACE regulations delineated in CFR 460.0 et al**. The Centers for Medicare and Medicaid Services (CMS) regularly promulgates guidance on these regulations and develops systems for auditing compliance with these regulations. PACE programs must also comply with prevailing state regulations and licensure since PACE is a three-way agreement between the PACE program, the federal government, and the state. Creating a "deep bench" with knowledge of the various regulations is a good strategy in PACE. For example, having team members steeped in Part D regulations is important. If a PACE program has not reached the point where these compliance resources are handled internally, there are several third-party administrators and other plan benefit manager (PBM) firms that provide these services on a contractual basis. Consultants can help achieve the "nirvana" of high-quality, regulatory compliance and financial success. Ultimately, it is up to the PACE leadership to identify where the expertise comes from—either it is internal to the organization, or it must be found externally.

PACE programs generally have access to a tremendous amount of data, including claims data. PACE leadership becomes the advocate for the data resources that the team needs to deliver on quality outcomes. This requires extensive work with information technology (IT) experts to develop systems to meet comprehensive needs. As PACE programs grow, demands for data reporting for compliance and analytics necessitate a move to more automated solutions. Frequently, when PACE programs begin, data can be managed on Excel spreadsheets or through a manual chart review. The recent change in the CMS audit protocols prompted many within PACE to rethink systems to automate the collection of their data into formats that CMS requires. PACE programs frequently use dashboards as a means of taking large volumes of data and putting them into a format that is accessible and actionable. Circulating weekly, monthly, and annual dashboards on utilization management are certainly important. Quality dashboards and trend analysis can be used to focus quality improvement programs. In terms of participant experience, analysis of grievance and safety events are important elements for leadership tracking. Effective PACE leaders frequently toggle between "never losing sight of the big picture" while being conversant enough in the details of this work to focus attention on what is critical. **Never underestimate the importance of transitioning raw data into useful, actionable information**.

Integration of Palliative Care

Palliative care is discussed in detail in another chapter of this book. A strong palliative care program requires organizational commitment articulated by its leader. As many hospice programs have entered the PACE community, there is a recognition of the vast expertise that is available in PACE to create stronger palliative programs. In addition, geriatricians and hospice/palliative-care-certified providers that have practiced in PACE for years are well equipped to provide the medical aspects of this care. Leaders also support the inclusion of other resources that are essential for meeting the whole-person needs of those in palliative care, including spiritual support. PACE programs have embraced the importance of palliative care for years, though it is sometimes known by other terms such as "comfort care" or "supportive care." The National PACE Association has convened a large work group to address how PACE can further integrate and enhance palliative care within the context of PACE. Creating systems and structures to support strong palliative care is a key task of a PACE leader. These include resources for education, competency training, and staffing. A commitment to measuring the quality of the palliative care program and constantly innovating to see it thrive is a cornerstone of PACE.

Garnering Resources

With reliance on a PACE Center as the hub of this model of care, access to capital for initial construction and future expansion is an important task of the PACE leader. Frequently, the resources for construction, or tenant improvements to existing buildings, come from the sponsoring organization or health system. There are also capital investment opportunities that can be accessed on the private market. PACE development has included construction projects that tap into a broad array of public and tax credit options. For example, through partnerships with the development of HUD 202 housing, a PACE Center can be created on the first floor of the housing complex. This can be an exciting, successful community-based option. PACE programs have also worked with their local cities and counties to fund development. Private non-for-profit foundations have also taken the lead in creating capital for PACE development. PACE leadership should always be thinking about capital needs for long-term planning. PACE capital needs also extend to the acquisition of vans for transportation and funding IT infrastructure. Philanthropy can also be used to augment capital funding efforts or create special funds for innovation in PACE. Again, the role of the leader to constantly be creating capital for innovation and growth cannot be underestimated.

Summary

Brené Brown, in her book entitled Daring Greatly, quoted Seth Godin as follows: "Leadership is scarce because few people are willing to go through the discomfort required to lead. This scarcity makes leadership valuable … It's uncomfortable to challenge the status quo. …. If you're not uncomfortable in your work as a leader, it's almost certain you're not reaching your potential as a leader." [5] Dr. Brown, a licensed clinical social worker by training, captured the notion of *Daring Greatly* with her reference to Teddy Roosevelt's quote about "showing up in the arena." Each day, PACE offers some new dimension to the arena. **The ability to live in ambiguity, to stand in the arena, and to engage others in the transformation of care are all hallmarks of PACE leadership**.

References

1. Wheatley MJ. Who Do We Choose to Be? Facing Reality, Claiming Leadership, Restoring Sanity. Oakland, CA: Berrett-Koehler Publishers, Inc.; 2017. p. 51.
2. National PACE association. PACE 2.0 west coast Collaborative Presentation 2019.
3. Gong, Jade and Fitzgerald, Peter. "PACE Programs Are Ready to Grow Exponentially" HEALTH PROGRESS www.chausa.org MARCH - APRIL 2019.
4. National Academy of Medicine, "Effective Care for High-Need Patients: Opportunities for Improving Outcomes, Value and Health," 2017. https://nam.edu/HighNeeds/.
5. Brown, Brene'. Daring Greatly. Avery, Penguin Random House. 2012. p. 211.

Chapter 6
Starting and Growing a PACE Program

Joan Kwiatkowski, Emily Drennan, and Victoria Parker

Starting and Growing a PACE Program

What drives an organization or group of individuals to take on the challenge of opening a PACE program? PACE fills an important gap in the long-term care continuum. This model does the following:

- Presents a new concept of community-based care that is less than nursing home care but more than typical community interventions
- Offers a risk-based and flexible financing model that encourages the best use of the right resources at the right time and in the right location of care
- Creates an alternative care model for high-risk individuals for whom the traditional models of health care do not work

As we consider the PACE model, we will address the unique challenges, opportunities, and conditions that a PACE program will encounter as it opens and grows. This section will review the possible ownership models, how to use a marketing and gap analysis to inform about the implementation process, and the business plan.

Opening a Pace Program

Mission, Vision, and Values

A future operator of a PACE program should appreciate the value of the model and believe that the mission of PACE will result in better care for some of their most vulnerable community members. A future operator of a PACE program

J. Kwiatkowski (✉) · E. Drennan · V. Parker
PACE Organization of Rhode Island, Providence, RI, USA
e-mail: jkwiatkowski@pace-ri.org; edrennan@pace-ri.org; vparker@pace-ri.org

M. K. McNabney (ed.), *Community-Based Integrated Care for Older Adults*,
https://doi.org/10.1007/978-3-031-05137-1_6

should believe in a team approach to care, in the financial flexibility allowed under PACE regulations, and, most of all, in the value this model brings to individuals. It is hard work to operate a program whose operating budget is "at risk" for all incurred costs that fluctuate with performance and has significant regulatory latitude. On Lok, the first PACE program in the country, was sponsored by a federally qualified health center (FQHC). As a result, many of the early PACE programs were established by community health centers or preexisting nonprofit health care systems. Today, a PACE program might be incorporated as a stand-alone nonprofit organization or owned by a for-profit investment firm. Regardless of the legal definition of the owner/operator, all of these entities should believe in the mission and value of PACE and must adhere to the same federal regulations.

In 2013, 91 PACE programs existed across the country. The majority of these programs were sponsored by hospital systems or community agencies, such as hospice agencies or elder care social service organizations. As of 2020, more than 120 PACE programs exist across the country, with more opening soon, thanks to a nationwide initiative referred to as PACE 2.0. Facilitated by the National PACE Association (NPA) and funded by the John A. Hartford Foundation, West Health, and the Commonwealth Fund, this initiative is designed to support existing PACE centers to grow their census. The PACE 2.0 framework recommended a number of marketing and growth strategies, which will be discussed in this chapter. We will start at the beginning: Who owns and operates the PACE program?

Owner/Operator Scenarios

Each owner/operator scenario will have different financing resources with which to establish a new program. Other differences will include accounting capabilities, internal staff capacity, influence over legislative and regulatory regulations, physical plant ownership, and governance structure.

A larger health system might be able to "lend" a physician to become the PACE medical director through a service contract, whereas a stand-alone program might have to directly hire a physician to fill this key role.[1] A hospital might have a lobbyist on retainer and can use this individual to advocate with the state for changes to the Medicaid State Plan or the establishment of a rate methodology. A collaborative action of community agencies might need to use more grassroots tactics to achieve the same goal. A PACE program could share administrative staff, like human resources, finance, and education, through an arrangement with the parent organization. Each of these examples brings its own opportunity and complexity. In short, the Centers for Medicare and Medicaid Services (CMS) requires a defined entity as the owner/operator of the PACE program. Defining the actual entity with chief authority is the first step in developing a new PACE program.

[1] Funded by the John A. Hartford Foundation, West Health, and the Commonwealth Fund.

If the organization is an existing entity, such as a hospital system or a long-term care network or even a community health center, the nature of the relationship between the new entity, PACE, and its "parent" should be defined in a contract. The existing national PACE community is comprised of generous professionals who will gladly share their experiences to help others avoid pitfalls and benefit from prudent decisions.

Before we discuss corporate ownership, we want to clarify an important distinction during start-up. If a state already has a PACE program, then the path to opening an additional program will be different than in a state where there is no preexisting PACE program. If the state has PACE programs, then an entity needs to validate that the market it intends to serve is available. States may restrict the number of programs that can serve a market (set of zip codes) or require an application to earn the right to serve a market. Your state's Medicaid program will have the answer to that question.

If a state does not have a preexisting PACE program, then the first step is to advocate with Medicaid for an amendment to the Medicaid State Plan allowing PACE as a Medicaid benefit. Additionally, the state would have to agree to be a party to the three-way provider agreement (the PACE program, CMS, and Medicaid). Without these two critical steps established, an entity cannot move ahead with an application to CMS to become a PACE program.

Growing a PACE program is complex. The selection of a corporate structure can go in two directions: it can further complicate the opening of a program and result in an administrative burden that risks financial success, or the structure can be supportive, consistent with the mission, and clear enough to launch a very successful program that meets its intended goals. We will now discuss the three legal structures currently used to establish PACE programs.

Scenario 1: Stand Alone PACE Program

If the entity is a new nonprofit organization, the entity must be sure to file the necessary applications with the state to incorporate. The process can be lengthy depending on the state's process for review. In order to proceed, steps that may be necessary include claiming an official name, filing articles of incorporation, applying for Internal Revenue Service (IRS) tax exemption, applying for state tax exemption, drafting bylaws, appointing a board of directors, holding a meeting of the board, and obtaining necessary permits and licensure. New entities should ask the Department of Business Regulations (or similar state agency) if PACE is considered an insurance company or managed care plan and therefore held to governing regulations. Most states do not define PACE as a managed care plan; they consider them adult day programs based on licensure. It is important to know early in the process because managed care plans must establish cash reserves that might be cost prohibitive. The new entity should research which state licenses it must apply for; adult day centers and home care are two of the most common. Some PACE programs are licensed as outpatient clinics, while other states do not require any license as they interpret the federal regulations to be sufficient as a means to oversee safety and compliance.

Once you have secured approval from the state to apply for federal designation as a PACE program and have completed all necessary state incorporation steps based on solid market and financial data, you are ready for the next step in establishing the actual program.

Scenario 2: PACE Program Owned by a Larger System

If the new PACE program is affiliated with a larger organization or being created through a collaboration of existing but separate agencies, all parties must clearly define governance and financial support. There is no worse time to discover a lack of financial support than during a financial crisis. To successfully open a PACE program, it is important to seek clarity regarding capital lending, bank financing, governance, and authority.

Some sponsoring or parent organizations lend capital to the PACE programs in the development phase. Sometimes this money is a contribution with no expectation of repayment, and sometimes the sponsoring agency wants the investment back in the form of payment over time. These terms should be clear as it is not uncommon for a PACE program to need 2–3 years before it becomes profitable. If repayment is required, then establish a budget and financial reporting system accordingly. Or if a PACE program can defer its obligation, then in a contract, define when and how the investment is to be repaid. There have been examples of PACE programs sponsored by coalitions and health systems where repayment was sought years into operation without a contractual obligation creating legal costs, and operational distractions.

If a sponsoring organization cannot or chooses not to provide all of the start-up capital, it can serve as a guarantor to a bank loan. In this example, the PACE program is taking out the loan, and the sponsoring organization will agree to guarantee repayment in the event the PACE program cannot meet its payment schedule or other covenants defined in the loan agreement. This arrangement is appealing to a sponsoring organization because it assumes no cash obligation upfront. The guarantee does need to be recognized in the organization's balance sheet, and sometimes funds might need to be placed in escrow, depending on the lender. To serve as a guarantor, the organization will likely have a strong governance role to protect its interest in the PACE program. As an example, one PACE program developed through a coalition of separate nonprofit entities was able to secure five of the entities to serve as guarantors. When the program repaid its debt to the bank, these organizations were released from their obligations. In the initial letters of agreement between the new PACE organization and these entities, it was clearly stated that at no time could the entities seek payment from PACE for its commitment. Their commitment guaranteed that they held one board seat and had veto power over issues such as refinancing, closure, or sale of the program.

Other areas of role confusion occur when there is a lack of definition with authority. What can PACE do on its own? Who has the final decision on the selection of vendors, contracting for services, or establishing employee benefits?

If the PACE executive director must defer to a board or governance committee and then needs to seek additional approval from hospital leadership, it should be clear up front. Many challenges arise in the early stages of opening a PACE program. You do not need to add to the challenges by questioning who has authority over which decision.

Some sponsorship arrangements include the use of the parent company's administrative services, e.g., accounting and information technology. While this can help a PACE program establish these functions quickly and efficiently, there can be downsides. First, PACE may not be a priority for these departments, resulting in a slower response time to requests or the staff not being adequately trained on the duties required for a risk-based, community service program. Reports might be late, electronic medical record systems designed for hospital or physicians' use might not lend themselves to the needs of a community program, or a general lack of understanding of PACE regulatory complexities might expose the PACE program to inconsistencies and survey issues. If the program is to use a parent's administrative services, prepare a written document that defines the expectations, roles, and intersection between the needs of the PACE program and the parent's abilities. A written document will spare you angst when leadership turns over and the new person's assumptions do not match the previous leader's intentions.

Scenario 3: For-Profit PACE Program

In 2018, CMS abolished its requirement that PACE programs must be nonprofit organizations [1]. There are a growing number of for-profit PACE programs either sponsored or owned by for-profit nursing home chains or investment firms. The investment firm's strategy is to buy multiple struggling programs in various markets anchored by one or two larger, strong programs. It is too early to tell what impact this change will have on competition, quality, and financial success. Ownership by an investment firm will likely require that profit be shared among its investors. Policy consultants and providers fear that allowing for profit ownership will result in a reduction in quality, more aggressive market competition, and a negative impact on PACE's reputation. There have been recent articles that examined the quality of care at large for-profit PACE providers. In one article [2], the writer interviewed staff who had previously been employed by this entity who reported that the focus on growth, the management of service requests and reduced staffing levels impacted quality and access to care. Additional studies are needed to better define the differences between for-profit and nonprofit PACE programs.

Regulatory Steps

State Approval and Partnership

A strong partnership with the state results in greater, long-term success. The state needs to understand how PACE operates so it can support the growth of the program.

Answering the following questions will help you to gauge whether your state will support PACE:

- What is the state budget for spending on long-term care support and services and on home and community-based services (HCBS)?
- What is your state's commitment to HCBS generally?
- Who on your team can manage the task of facilitating the application/licensing process? And what is their relationship to key state program staff?
- Is there an existing state PACE trade association that can assist you in establishing a relationship with key state partners?

For the purposes of this discussion, we will assume that the state supports the opening of a new PACE program. The next steps are to complete the federal application. The state must submit a letter of support and a rate-setting methodology as part of your application. The state must agree to sign a three-way contract between itself, CMS, and PACE. Given that there is work to be done by the state, you should be confident in its support so you can get the required application materials necessary to submit a successful application.

PACE Application

The application process is well defined on both the national PACE website [3] and the CMS website. Most organizations hire a technical assistance consultant to assist in completing the application. Some programs need up to 2 years to complete the application. The process is time-consuming because you must submit a business plan, an organizational chart, policies and procedures, and many other supporting documents. Many programs experience challenges along the way, which further delay submission, such as a change in state leadership that may not support a new program, state budget cuts, and parent organization changes. A well-organized, experienced consultant is money well spent toward the completion of an efficient and successful process.

Financing

We recommend that several analyses be completed early in the process to confirm the need, cost, and sustainability of a new program. These include initial investment, business plan, market analysis, and risk management plan.

Initial Investment

At the time of this writing, start-up costs for a new PACE center averaged $3–5 million. The initial investment will depend on several factors. Some questions to think about are as follows:

- Is there an existing site that can be used for the PACE center?
- Are there existing staff employed by a parent corporation whose salaries are funded through that entity, or are they funded by PACE?
- Are there grants available to offset any start-up expenses?
- What is the bank loan or financing structure that will support the cost of the start-up?

New PACE programs are spending money before receiving any revenue. CMS requires that staff be hired and ready to provide services before the first enrollee crosses your threshold. The business plan should account for these expenses. If you assume a 2-year approval process and a slow start-up phase, your costs could easily exceed the $3–5 million quoted earlier. Market variability plays a huge role as well. One PACE program received considerable state funds to open, while another received seed money from foundations to cover the start-up phase. Know your costs upfront and create a sound income stream to cover those costs because you will not be receiving income from revenue for quite some time.

Business Plan

A business plan is not a market analysis. You will need a market analysis as a part of your business plan. The business plan is intended to establish financial goals. It will tie together the results of the market and gap analyses, allowing you to attach cost estimates and numbers, i.e., staffing ratios. Many organizations hire consultants to assist with this task. There are several well-established consultants with a national presence who have PACE expertise.

The business plan will include financial projections based on census growth. Most PACE programs establish an 18-month budget as a starting point. The first 2–4 months may rightfully indicate a slow climb in the census. If the program is new to the market, it will take time to create a successful enrollment message and have consumers understand the value of the program. In contrast to a slow start, you could experience a successful start and then watch census drag after 6 months of operation. This pattern represents a pent-up demand and a reaction from marketing and communication efforts. Once that initial burst ends, you might find a lag before more consistent enrollment patterns are established. Many PACE programs begin with one enrollee—do not be surprised if that is your experience.

A business plan can be a useful tool in the planning process. The document should lay out the path of growth. You are required to have a certain number of staff hired before the doors open. The business plan will educate you on how long you can sustain the expenses before you open the doors. The business plan can be useful in the establishment of contract rates, the selection of vendors, the timing of hires, and the determination of your greatest risk during the first months of operation. The other key questions and components of a business plan can be found below.

Key questions and components of a business plan
Finance
How are you financing the start-up of the PACE program (assume anywhere between $2–5 million)? Lenders or investors? What are the terms and repayment obligations?
Who is the parent corporation, and what is its contribution?
Will additional funding be needed? If so, by who?
Cash flow needs—remember that you need to be fully staffed and equipped prior to gaining CMS approval to operate
Grants or donations that can offset start-up costs account for grants and donations only after you have received the support; some states have provided grants to new PACE programs as a way to encourage the growth of the model. Some PACE programs have received foundation funding to pay for upfront costs or secure a location. Grants and donations reduce the financial losses the program will inevitably experience in its early days of operations
At what point is a financial breakeven anticipated?
What will be the rate of return when the program is fully established? In other words, what is the sweet spot of enrollment that will make you financially stable?
What other services might you consider as a reimbursement option? For example, PACE programs that provide traditional adult day care. What is the sweet spot of payer mix to make the program financially viable?
What does it cost to fully equip a day center?
Staffing and organization
What does a fully staffed PACE program look like? What is the staffing requirement for a start-up, and what does that cost?
Consider the organizational structure, leadership, and key staff
Who will sustain the overall development of the program?
Who are the clinical leaders that provide support for the program?
Do you have an accounting system that supports billing and reporting?
Do you have experience with quality assurance/reporting?
How will you introduce the PACE model, including the importance of the IDT, to those who staff the program?

Market Analysis

It is critical to include solid market data in your business plan. This data should include statewide demographics (age, income, density) and be drilled down to specific communities the program intends to serve. A market analysis is an examination of the population that lives within a specific market or area, including information such as their age, their income, their housing status, access to health care, the types of health care available within a market, and access to transportation. It is a study on how well a market is resourced. As it relates to PACE, a market analysis will focus on health status and access to care.

"Know your data" should be your mantra throughout the opening phase. We recommend hiring a competent consultant who can complete a thorough market analysis early in your planning process. It can take from 3 months to 2 years to open a PACE program after you get the initial state approval. Because of the extended time, many changes can occur in the industry, in your state, and in the preferred market, causing you to rethink, restructure, or stop the project altogether. Retest the market throughout the opening process so you can build specific enrollment tactics that can easily pivot, garnering the best results quickly. This section provides a breakdown of the market analysis, including key questions that would be helpful to consider during the opening process.

There are three ingredients to a solid market analysis: knowing the *market size*, learning the *availability of alternative services* (sometimes called "look-alikes"), and *gap analysis* or determining what is NOT available to seniors.

Market Size

Market size will tell you what the demand for the PACE service is. You will learn important characteristics about older adults who live in the market you are serving. Understanding your market size will help you develop your potential for enrollment and growth in participants. Looking beyond what is current in the market and what the market will look like in 5 years is important to consider. Questions to consider asking are the following:

- How many Medicaid or dual-eligible clients are there in your market area currently? In 5 years?
- How many older adults match the level of care your state views as eligible for PACE?
- Population size of those 50+, 65+, 75+, 85+ in zip codes—how many of those in that age range are living with disability? What are their main diagnoses?
- What is the size of the population in the above age range with income below Medicaid financial eligibility?
- Of the defined population, how many are nursing home eligible?

Availability of Service Alternatives

Understanding the services and programs that exist in your market can help you adjust your marketing strategy and build referral networks. It can also paint a picture of the success and challenges of other organizations that serve a similar population profile. Competitors of PACE in your market could include Medicare advantage plans, state waiver programs, community health centers, and other provider networks. Questions to consider asking are as follows:

- How many competitors or look-alike programs are there in your market? Managed care penetration in your market?
- What is the anticipated threat of additional competitors to move into the market share?
- What is the financial and clinical eligibility requirement for a Medicaid-funded community-based care option?

- What are the regulatory limitations on the size/growth of Medicaid-funded community-based care?
- What is the current capacity of other community-based care options in your service area? How many are there? How many people can they serve (beds)? What is the cost to consumer? Quality reputation? Enrollment demand? Has their enrollment changed overtime?

Analyze the results of the data collection process. If done thoroughly, the market analysis should clarify the likelihood of success and sustainability.

Gap Analysis

A gap analysis is determining what people do not have access to in a market. A gap analysis might be included in a market study, or it might be a separate exercise used to determine if and when to expand services. This specific activity is particularly useful when arguing a position for a grant or expanded funding. A gap analysis may include the following comparisons.

Comparisons	What will it tell you?
The number of older adults living in a particular service area compared to the number of primary care providers, transportation services, home care services available for a Medicaid population, dental services, etc.	The current landscape of providers that are available to the population of older adults living in the service area; if the service area under review already has several primary care providers and adult day centers, PACE may not want to pick that service area as the central location
The socioeconomic status of older adults compared to the housing options in that part of the state	If there is only private-assisted living available but the socioeconomic status is low for older adults living in that service area, then they need a provider that meets the needs of the socioeconomic group
The workforce challenges in your market compared to the sufficient staffing needed for a PACE program	If the workforce challenge is a shortage of certified nursing assistants and no support from the state, i.e., training programs for potential CNAs, then you may need to consider contracting with a home health agency to fill that need
The existing opportunities to establish community partnerships compared to the ability of your program to outsource services like transportation and home care	Like the workforce challenge above, if you know that there is a need to outsource and contract with other agencies for service needs, then what is your capacity to do so? The program will need a contract associate who can negotiate contracts with potential vendors and perform oversight duties of these relationships
The potential location of your building compared to the ability of your program to provide services	Once you have a potential location in mind, you will need to ensure that it will not cost the organization significant money to provide services. For example, you will need to know the potential mileage the PACE van will be driving to reach participants and bring them back and forth to the day center. You will not want the day center to be in one corner of the state if all the participants live in the opposite corner

Experienced PACE leaders will tell you that they retest their market assumptions regularly. The results dictate marketing strategies, enrollment tactics, vendor partnerships, and more. This section could be a book on its own merits. We hope we have provided enough details and explanations to start a successful planning process.

Risk Management

You have state support to open a PACE program. Your market, gap, and business analyses support the opening of a program. Now, how are you going to successfully operate and manage the risk inherent in a capitated financing model?

PACE is an insurance product. Therefore, you must have early warning systems in place to mitigate and control the risk. You must have data management systems and health plan management strategies in place. A new PACE program worked so hard to open that it missed the need to register for a critical CMS portal, leaving it without federal revenue for 6 months.

Here are some examples of what a risk management system would track:

- Data dashboard, which includes the utilization of services, such as nursing home placements, hospitalizations, emergency room (ER) usage, readmissions, medication types and costs, etc.
- Trend data on referral activity, unanticipated disenrollments, and successful marketing tactics
- Risk score and dropped hierarchical condition category reports to validate that all of the participants' health conditions are accurately documented and their risk score reflects their acuity
- Vendor performance, such as cancellation rates of home care providers, which then result in ER visits or readmission rates to hospitals

The next section will cover contracting with vendors for services. Paying vendors can be complicated. If you are owned by a health system, the system might see PACE as a way to balance losses in other programs. If the PACE program is incorporated as a stand-alone entity, then you pay accurately and within reason, compared to market, state, and/or federal rate, to stabilize your financial performance. The details matter when determining vendor rates.

A PACE program will contract with a variety of providers, which will deliver clinical services to its participants. Depending on how a PACE program is defined in state statute or the Medicaid State Plan, the program may be justified in paying Medicaid rates to vendors. Most programs pay using the Medicare fee schedules for relevant services (e.g., consulting a physician or hospital admission) and Medicaid fees for covered benefits (e.g., nursing home custodial bed or adult day rates). Over time, a PACE program learns more about the cost of care in its region, the general needs of its participants, and the risk factors that can threaten financial stability. Use trend data to track these factors. The trend data will tell you when and how to adjust practices (e.g., too many cardiology consults or too many brand prescription medications versus generic) and control costs.

Some PACE programs pay Medicare, plus a percent of cost, while still others implement quality incentives to encourage particular outcomes (e.g. a quality incentive to a home care vendor who meets call out or cancellation targets). PACE can apply federal quality incentives when contracting with providers. Understand that you have latitude when it comes to what you pay and how to pay so you shape not only the financial future you want but also the delivery and services your participants need.

One seemingly unrelated yet key issue for PACE programs is paying attention to when Medicaid and Medicare increase provider rates and how the timing of this activity aligns with your own rate setting timeline with the state. In one state, the rate of the PACE program was reviewed every 3 years. Over that 3-year period, Medicaid doubled its payment to home care vendors and transportation services. Because the PACE program's contracts with home care and transportation vendors are based on Medicaid rates, they had to increase their payments without any additional dollars to their own rate to cover that increase. Three years later, the program's rate was increased accordingly, but they had to cover those increases for three years.

Risk management means managing your data so you can pivot behavior quickly to avoid downside risk. For example, a team should be aware that it is admitting more participants to nursing homes for custodial placement. The reimbursement received by the PACE program does not usually equal or exceed the Medicaid bed rate. Give the teams financial and utilization data so they are aware of the consequences of their decisions. They still might place an individual because that is the best decision for that individual, and they will know the cost implication for the program. That is the PACE model in action—flexibility to do what is necessary and the financial knowledge to understand the consequences.

Many PACE programs secure a reinsurance policy. This policy insures the program against losses associated with extremely high costs usually associated with hospitalizations. These policies can be a lifesaver for a young program whose staff is still learning how to be a team. Some policies cover long stays or expensive hospital costs and subacute costs. Read the fine print. Some policies cover within a calendar year only (so an admission in December with a discharge in January is not covered) or up to a specific dollar amount, which does not include medication costs. With time, you will understand which policy best mitigates the risks the team, the community, and the participants face.

Suffice it to say that data is king. Your market, what the risk scores are, how much you spend—you need to know it all. Developing a data system that can compile, analyze, and disseminate data to the team and managers is a worthwhile investment. As you are building your operating systems and workflow, be sure to create a data and information management system that will keep everyone informed. A well-informed team will make prudent decisions that best serve both the participants and the program.

Growing a Pace Program

The PACE Message and Explaining to the Public

Once you find the potential participants, you must explain to them and their caregivers why the PACE model is the best choice for their physical, mental, and social needs. Since the model is complex and new, it is important to discuss key components of joining PACE. Three main messages to communicate are as follows:

1. Once enrolled, the participant will use PACE as their primary care provider.
2. PACE will become the insurance provider for this person, and there is a potential for a cost share associated with their enrollment in PACE.
3. The participant has access to a number of service providers (the 11-member interdisciplinary team), which they will be expected to meet with on a regular basis for care planning assessments. The care plan will be established based on participant goals.

A potential barrier to enrollment for many PACE participants is changing their primary care provider from their community doctor to PACE. For some individuals, they may have seen their primary care provider in the community for over 20 years and feel very comfortable with that relationship. It is likely that the person also has many chronic illnesses and is comfortable with how their current providers care for them. Just like any other insurance company, patients will be required to utilize providers that are in network for their care. PACE can best manage someone's care when it has direct oversight and medical decision-making authority. Without this, it would be sharing the risk of someone's care with a provider that is outside of network. To avoid the potential barrier to enrollment, PACE does allow new enrollees to see their community doctor once a year and often contracts with out-of-network providers to ensure continuity of care. Most participants see the value in PACE providing their medical services and stop seeing their community doctor soon after joining.

For PACE Rhode Island (RI), 94% of participants are dual eligible, meaning they utilize Medicare (65+) and Medicaid (low income). Some potential enrollees could be connected to a Medicare Advantage plan, a prescription assistance program, veterans' benefits, private insurance, etc. Health insurance is complicated, and it can be difficult to explain to a potential enrollee that they will now be insured by PACE as opposed to their usually insurance carrier. Some individuals may be apprehensive to give up their existing benefits.

Potential enrollees may be concerned with their cost of care. In the example above, where 94% of the PACE participants are dual eligible (Medicare and Medicaid beneficiaries), it means that 94% of the individuals enrolled in PACE-RI have no cost associated with the care they receive. It means the enrollee will never see copayment or monthly premium or meet a deductible to receive their care. The program may be perceived as a service provider for dual-eligible individuals only. That is simply not true. Anyone can enroll in PACE from any socioeconomic group. The cost share for PACE services will be determined based on the individual's income. If someone is not eligible for their state Medicaid allowance, there will be a cost share, which will be paid each month. This would be similar to an insurance premium, which is paid on a monthly basis.

There are many ways to explain the cost-share determination. If a potential enrollee is going to have a cost share, it may be helpful to review the individual's income and understand their current premiums and out-of-pocket expenses. Once you determine the individual's monthly expenses under their current insurance, compare that cost to what the PACE cost-share amount is. The PACE cost share also covers all care and services needed for the individual to maintain their independence within the community, which includes the full coverage of things, like medication, hearing aids, supplies, and reading glasses.

The care team is the third component of the PACE model to be explained to potential participants and those involved in their care. For some individuals enrolling, they may not have had access to the type of care and wrap-around services that PACE is able to provide. The services are determined based on the care team's assessment, medical necessity, and ability to maintain safety in the community. This concept will be important for new enrollees to understand so that their expectations of the services they are eligible to receive are realistic.

PACE is designed to blend medical and social care, which allows older adults to maintain their independence in the community. PACE is not an option for older adults or caregivers who are seeking long-term care placement. It will be crucial in the explanation of the PACE model to ensure the understanding of the partnership, which is required to make PACE a successful option for healthy aging.

Marketing

Staffing

When PACE programs start out, they are more likely to hire a marketing professional in the community who will take on certain marketing campaigns and measure their effectiveness. As the organization grows and becomes more sophisticated, you will want to staff your own marketing department. The staff within the marketing department could include but is not limited to an experienced marketing professional in a leadership position, communications, graphic design, development, and public relations. The marketing staff will work closely with the intake and enrollment staff because one of the goals of marketing is to drive inquiries and enrollment to PACE. If you are an organization attached to a larger system, there is potential to share the marketing staff of the larger system as a resource to create and track your marketing materials.

Marketing Assessment

Once you begin reaching out to the community and enrolling participants, you will need to complete a marketing assessment. This is different than the marketing analysis you completed to open the program. You could hire a consultant to do this or utilize internal staff. The marketing assessment will help you understand if the efforts you are making toward enrollment are giving you the outcomes you want. For example, if your marketing analysis showed you that the highest number of older adults with significant health needs reside in specific zip codes, are your current marketing efforts focused on that part of the state? If yes, is the information you are marketing to those zip codes actually getting to older adults or caregivers? Is it prompting them to inquire about PACE services?

Essentially, the marketing assessment is needed to measure the effectiveness of your marketing materials. The assessment could include a complete review of all marketing collateral, including brochures, annual reports, and newsletters. Other marketing materials could include digital advertising, commercials, social media, website, and more. Many programs leverage grassroots events to market their program. Any opportunity to showcase the program is a good one and could be used as a key marketing strategy to help increase referrals and enrollment. Most programs have found that "seeing PACE in action" has a greater impact on referral sources, so tours are highly encouraged.

There are several things you can track to measure the success of your marketing program and gauge the level of brand awareness.

Metric	What it tells you
Number and duration of website visits	How effective your website is in keeping people engaged, where people are spending most of their time on the website
Number of inquiries and referrals	Whether or not the messaging of PACE is reaching people in the community
Percentage of inquiries and referrals that turn into enrollments	Whether or not the messaging of PACE is reaching the RIGHT people in the community, who will choose to enroll, not every inquiry will be an enrollment
Community surveys	An awareness of the general public's perception of the PACE program
Mystery shopper phone calls to potential referral sources	Whether the potential referral source is aware of PACE and if yes, understands the program and therefore would easily identify potential referrals for the PACE program

Marketing Strategies

Using a video technique to explain the PACE model is effective because it helps paint a visual picture of what the day center and other services look like. PACE commercials are most effective when using actual participants and real staff to show the emotional connection. Your marketing assessment will lead you to pinpoint the exact time of the day and station(s) that the commercial should air. If older adults are only watching television between the hours of 8 a.m. and 2 p.m., then the commercial should air at that time.

An increasingly important marketing tactic is the use of social media, including Facebook, Instagram, and LinkedIn. The information you market to these platforms could draw different audiences. Remember that marketing is important not only for census growth but also for the growth of your workforce, supporters in the community, and potential donors. By sharing a staff spotlight on Facebook or Instagram, you are showing that you are an organization that values your staff's contributions and, therefore, attracting potential employees to your page. You could use LinkedIn as a resource to share open positions or innovative partnerships with other local businesses. If you find that the social media efforts are working for their intended purpose, then it will be important to continue implementing these strategies. Fatigue in advertising is not allowed. The program will lose momentum, costing the program a consistent stream of inquiries and enrollments. The momentum is costly and time-consuming to rebuild.

Another great resource for PACE marketing is the PACE website. You can link the PACE website to posts you are making on social media, you can mention it in the videos you create, and you can spotlight it in your print materials. A strong PACE website will include a homepage that explains the PACE model with common and easy-to-understand phrases and eye-catching graphics. The website should have a PACE eligibility section that explains how to enroll. It may be prudent to include an eligibility quiz directly on your website. You are able to track analytic information about the people who visit your website, like how long they stay on each page and where the most clicks happen. If you notice in your marketing assessment that most clicks on your website are on the "open positions" page and not on the eligibility section, then you would know that most people visiting the website are looking to work at PACE rather than enroll.

Relationships are key to successful marketing. Relationships can occur at all levels of the organization. The intake and enrollment staff, the marketing staff, those staff who work closely with vendors and all staff should establish positive working relationships with community representatives. PACE programs vary in how they recognize supporting referral sources. Sending a plate of cookies or honoring people at annual meetings are allowed, but taking everyone out for an expensive meal is not. Be sure your tactics are within regulatory bounds.

While there are many opportunities to market PACE, the most fulfilling marketing tactic is word of mouth, whether it is participants recommending their family, friends, and loved ones or your workforce referring neighbors and companions. A good measure of your program's success and opportunity to grow is if the participants and workforce are recommending its growth to others.

Referral Sources

The results of the marketing assessment will direct your outreach efforts. You are the new service provider that specializes in geriatric care—you have to be where older adults are. Strategic referral networks could include hospital case managers and discharge teams, community health workers employed by local community action programs or community health centers, churches, resident service coordinators or building staff of senior housing, community day and senior centers, other managed care programs, emergency management folks, i.e., police, fire personnel, ambulance, emergency medical technicians (EMT). This list goes on.

PACE is a program that specializes in caring for high-risk and high-maintenance older adults, making it appealing for community providers to refer patients to the PACE program. A good marketing strategy with hospital case managers or discharge planners includes education, provision of marketing materials and easy access to PACE enrollment staff. If hospital discharge teams recognize the same older adult coming in and out of the hospital multiple times, then that individual may be a good fit for PACE so that they can receive the coordinated care they need. The intake team that works to onboard participants should make strong relationships with case managers and discharge planners for this to be successful.

If the program you have established is owned or operated by a larger system, like a community health center or hospital, then the referral network between providers may be easier to establish and maintain. For example, if the owner of the community health center is the same owner as the PACE program attached to it, then it would be in the owner's best interest to refer patients of the health center to the PACE program and keep them within network. Clear communication to the health center about growth projections and census demands will be important to maintain to ensure that the PACE staff is not onboarding more participants than it is capable of caring for. Alternatively, if it is within the PACE program's strategic plan to grow but the health center it is attached to is not providing the in-network referral, then there need to be clear conversations that lead to mission alignment for both entities. We know from experience that most health systems do not refer to their own PACE program, partly due to communication breakdown and partly due to control issues. Within a health care system, each unique program is held to individual financial metrics. Referrals across programs may not prove financially advantageous and make it hard to meet the financials goals.

Churches are a hub for community events of all ages, so it is no surprise that we find individuals attending church well into their old age. Churches provide relief to those who may be struggling, including caregivers who could be caring for potential PACE participants. You will want to ensure that you have marketing materials available and relationships with churchgoers in the community. PACE has been successful in cultivating strong relationships with religious orders.

Resident service coordinators (RSCs) are individuals who work in low-income housing, senior housing, or community housing and manage the day-to-day operations and safety of the residents in the building. Their job is extremely important, and there are not nearly enough of them. RSCs rely on programs like PACE to keep their residents safe and in their housing for as long as possible. This profession does see high levels of turnover, so constant communication and reeducation are needed. PACE can be a solution for resident service coordinators who need to ensure their residents are able to continue living in their homes. In addition to the resident service coordinator, housing complexes typically employ a maintenance or cleaning person who helps ensure the safety of the building. Maintenance and cleaning employees may witness older adults who need more assistance than they are able to provide within the housing complex. That is where PACE can be an option.

Other community workers and volunteers are sources for referral to PACE. Some programs have established partnerships with ambulance companies, emergency medical technicians (EMT), police officers, etc. Older adults in the community may not be aware of the services provided by PACE and rely on EMTs and police officers for their safety in the community. When these professionals receive multiple phone calls from older individuals or have contact with older adults who appear to be in need, they may be able to connect them to a provider like PACE.

There are many other referral networks that can be established to encourage PACE enrollment. By using communication strategies and establishing relationships, you will see enrollment grow. In addition to your outreach efforts, people in the community will begin inquiring directly. The most common referral source for PACE-RI is word of mouth (participants referring participants) and partnerships with local community health centers.

Competitors Serving Similar Populations

While other community day and senior centers may feel like a competition to the PACE program, they can be utilized as a referral network. When older adults who attend day centers are no longer able to maintain attendance due to their worsening medical conditions, the senior center director may only refer that individual to a nursing home because they feel that is where they would be the safest. If the senior center director understood the PACE model and knew of its existence, then they would be able to refer their day center attendees. You cannot assume that community day and senior centers are going to know and understand the PACE model. Some senior centers are run by a municipality, some are volunteer driven, and some are privately owned. The levels of understanding and willingness to refer may vary among sites. Constant communication is necessary to ensure a mutual understanding of each other's capabilities.

As states continue to rebalance long-term care, other managed care programs will continue to enter the market. The individuals in the community who are eligible for managed care programs could be the same individuals who are eligible for PACE enrollment. Again, managed care could be seen as a potential competitor but could also be a potential referral agent for PACE. As managed care enrollees become more complex and riskier to care for, it may be in their best interest to refer the individual to PACE, where their care can be provided more effectively. In Rhode Island, we found managed care companies were eager to establish a referral relationship with PACE. The managed care companies readily admitted their inability to provide intensive services and home-based interventions, leaving them financially vulnerable.

Enrollment and Growth

Once you have secured state approval, financing, licensure, and staff, you need to plan out your enrollment and onboarding processes. These elements are vital to have in place before opening to help make the progression from inquiry to PACE enrollment as smooth as possible for your potential participants.

Enrollment: The Intake Process

The establishment of a comprehensive intake assessment form can assist the enrollment team during the intake process. The intake form should consist of information specific to the potential enrollee, like demographics, social history, a list of current diagnoses and medications, and questions regarding the person's ability to perform activities of daily living (ADLs) and instrumental activities of daily living (IADLs). The intake assessment should also include a designated form that the person can sign to release medical records to the providers. The intake form should also include questions about those who may or may not be responsible for the individual's safety. This would include questions about primary contacts, who may be involved in the person's care, what type of support the person currently needs, and what type of support the person currently has. The intake form will be approved during the CMS approval process. CMS will guide you if the form does not meet regulatory intent. The form can be customized and include unique details about your program. We advise you to ask the IDT members what key elements they need to know early in the intake process and include those questions in the intake form.

The staff who completes the intake assessments will be required to meet with participants in the home setting. They need to be well versed in the PACE model, respectful of the diverse home environments, be able to establish appropriate professional boundaries with families, be able to manage the expectations of service provision, and be curious enough to ask the right questions to understand the participants' needs. The enrollment staff will need to communicate the outcomes of the intake assessment to the care team so that when the potential participant enrolls, the clinical staff understands their needs as well. The team can decide to initiate additional assessments for any onboarding participant.

The enrollment staff person needs to paint a complete picture of the potential enrollee. This means that if an enrollment staff member sees that knobs are missing on the stove but the potential enrollee explains that they are fully capable of cooking three meals a day, then there is a discrepancy between what the person is telling you and what is actually happening in their home. Another example could be that the enrollment staff person notices an enormous number of dishes in the sink and food left out but the person explains that they are fully capable of cleaning their home. The more information and insight the enrollment team can gain before someone enrolls, the more prepared the team will be to provide the right care.

When an intake assessment is completed, the participant will need a medical assessment performed by a primary care provider. The medical assessment, in conjunction with the intake assessment, and the necessary required documents needed to obtain financial eligibility will be submitted to the state for approval. The state will approve the individual's level of care (needs to meet the nursing home level of care, or in Rhode Island, the leveling system should be high or the highest to be eligible for PACE). The level of care is determined by state officials, typically nurses, who review the assessments in the application and identify the official level. If a participant does not meet the required level of care, it is a learning opportunity for your staff to better screen potential enrollees. In addition, it is an opportunity to offer education to the state officials determining the level so that they have a better understanding of what the PACE model can offer. The additional documents submitted will determine their financial eligibility, which will identify the potential cost share. The approval process can take anywhere from 14 to 90 days. Encouraging the state to develop a prompt approval process is key early in the life of a program. Each enrollment matters in reaching financial goals.

Onboarding Participants

Once approval is communicated back to the PACE program by the state, the PACE IDT will review the completed assessments and establish an interim care plan that will include the anticipated services needed for the new participant. A final enrollment conference will be scheduled where the participant obtains their PACE insurance card and the interim care plan and signs official enrollment documents. PACE enrollment always begins on the first of the month. At that point, PACE will be responsible for the provision of all care and services.

The onboarding of participants requires an enormous amount of internal and external communication. The IDT needs a strong understanding of the participant enrolling—what services are needed and who will provide them. The participant needs to understand their enrollment into PACE—when they should stop seeing external providers, when they will start seeing PACE providers, and, if applicable, attending the PACE day center. The state partner needs to communicate the approval of the participant's eligibility, so streamlining a process with the state partner and maintaining a strong relationship is a necessity.

Physical Space

The PACE center is the central hub of activity where anything from socialization and sharing meals to medical oversight and collaboration can take place in real time under one roof (see Chap. 9). A benefit of the PACE model is care coordination. One of the reasons why the 11-member interdisciplinary team is able to coordinate care efficiently is because all providers on the team are able to collaborate in the same building. The layout of the PACE center allows all disciplines to connect and communicate with each other effectively. At PACE-RI, the registered nurse and social worker assigned to a single caseload of participants physically share an office to increase communication. The physical layout of a PACE center typically includes a day and health center model with a rehab room attached.

Day Center

Participants are assigned a day center attendance schedule based on medical necessity and their interest in attendance (see Chap. 9). There is a range of activities that happen in the day center, such as card games, BINGO, men's/women's group, technology classes, music, and entertainment. The day center is staffed by certified nursing assistants, recreational therapists, and a day center director. A day center nurse is available to participants throughout the day for any issues that require clinical attention. The day center is a place where staff can physically see participants and interact with them for formal assessments or informal greetings and conversations. Relationship building happens in the day center among staff and participants and also between participants, making it a great opportunity for socialization to occur. In the annual participant satisfaction survey done at PACE-RI, we have found that the day center experience consistently ranks highest in terms of overall satisfaction. Participants report feeling a sense of purpose when they attend the day center.

Transportation

PACE provides transportation to participants attending the day center and to all medical appointments within the PACE center and to external providers (see Chap. 13). The transportation service is crucial to the care of older adults in the community. Often, transportation can be a barrier for older individuals who no longer drive and lack caregiver support for rides. PACE is able to offer a specialized, trusted service for participants, which is coordinated for them. The PACE program utilizes its own fleet of passenger vans and often contracts with local ambulance companies to transport participants. Contracted agencies have the ability to bring participants to the center on a stretcher for those who require that type of service. The transportation department is staffed by drivers, transport aides, a dispatcher, and a transportation manager.

Health Center (Medical Clinic)

The health center is attached to the day center, making it possible for participants attending the day center to see their primary care provider after enjoying a card game or a meal at lunch (see Chap. 9). The health center includes exam rooms, a medication room, supplies and storage, and medical records. The health center is staffed by an administrative assistant/scheduler, primary care providers (medical doctor (MD), registered nurse practitioner (RNP)), medical assistants, a medical record clerk, a medical coder, and a health center manager. Registered nurses may also work within the health center to assist with further coordination or hospital discharge planning. Participants are seen in the health center for a minimum of every 6 months for care planning assessments. Some PACE programs have implemented patient portals to allow participants and caregivers easy access to records.

Regulatory Awareness and Compliance

Key Processes and Methods

Since PACE is an insurance company, it is important to implement strong health plan management techniques early on. Competent health plan management will set the groundwork for a successful program. Some PACE programs deploy entire departments, typically led by a senior leader of quality and compliance, that oversee all regulatory requirements from CMS and other licensing bodies. Some of those requirements include level II reporting, facilitation of a quality committee, and audit preparation.

Health plan management begins with strong and clear policies and procedures. A PACE program uses a policy software system that tracks when revisions have been done, can send out updates to staff, and can send out affirmation documentation that requires staff to read and affirm a new policy. Audits are a second key element built as a means to ensure compliance with policies and procedures. Establishing an audit system involves creating a list of required activities, noting the source of where the activity is documented, creating an audit template, training staff to audit, and maintaining a calendar of audits, along with a process to disseminate the audit results. Below is a list of elements commonly reviewed in an audit system:

- Signed notes by providers, which ensure providers have closed out all notes in the electronic medical record (EMR)
- Services documented that match the goals in the care plan
- Grievances
- Falls
- Submission of CMS reports on time, complete and accurate
- Financial audits
- Pharmacy: drug utilization and documented evidence of diagnosis to support prescription

A third element is a communication plan. Establish a system by which audit results or changes in the policy are relayed to your staff. How does your team know they are out of compliance? Here is a list of possible ways programs can communicate their results to the staff:

- Creating a data dashboard that is available on a shared drive
- Posting quality and audit results on bulletin boards in the staff lounge
- Creating departmental standing agenda items that include these measures

- Integrating results into a quality committee, risk management committee, or utilization management committee
- Creating a data comic book that uses illustration as one means of education for the staff at all reading levels and language capabilities

A final element in a strong health plan management program is acting to improve outcomes. You have set the expectation, you have audited for results, you have shared the results, and now you need to see improvement or action. Use the compliance program or quality staff to move a plan of action forward.

Health plan management is focused on your obligations as an insurer. The tasks might differ, but the process is not different from developing a sound compliance program and an impressive quality program. *Compliance* addresses corporate compliance obligations and monitoring for issues, like fraud, government audits, governance, and legal behavior. A *quality program* will evaluate for good care, satisfaction, an educated workforce, and performance improvement opportunities. When used in conjunction, health plan management strategies, compliance policies, and quality initiatives can manage risk and encourage innovation.

Summary

In this chapter, the focus has been on the multilevel considerations for opening and growing a PACE organization. You have learned the various corporate structures of a program and have a sense of how each structure operates. You understand the importance of relationships across all sectors—with state officials, with community organizations, etc. You have a sense of the difference between market analysis and a business plan and the strategies for each. You have heard the recommendations to leverage marketing operations for a dynamic approach to recruiting participants. You know the intake process. Opening and growing a program requires the knowledge and understanding of the regulatory requirements. Furthermore, an individual who wishes to open and grow a PACE program needs to align with the overall mission of PACE. With persistency, curiosity, compassion, and grit, a leader will be successful at achieving both tasks.

References

1. Report to congress: the centers for medicare & medicaid services' evaluation of for-profit PACE programs under section 4804(b) of the balanced budget act of 1997. U.S. Department of Health and Human Services. 2015. https://innovation.cms.gov/files/reports/rtc_for-profit_pace_report_to_congress_051915_clean.pdf.
2. InnovAge: regulators, former employees raise quality of care concerns at company's PACE facilities. The Capitol Forum, 2021, pp. 9–12.
3. National PACE Association's. www.npaonline.org. Accessed Feb 16, 2022.

Chapter 7 The State's Role in the Implementation of PACE

James Pezzuti and Judith Baskins

Introduction

Congress passed legislation authorizing the Programs of All-Inclusive Care for the Elderly (PACE) to become a permanent provider under Medicare and Medicaid in 1997 and published the first PACE regulations in 1999. As part of those initial regulations, the Centers for Medicare & Medicaid Services (CMS) articulated their expectations for the role of states in the development and ongoing operations of PACE programs.

States have played a significant role in the development of PACE demonstration projects as well as other community-based alternatives to institutionalization. Most states have implemented home and community-based programs to provide comprehensive coordinated services to various groups of Medicaid recipients. As a result, states have gained extensive experience in demographic analysis and contracting with entities that are capable of delivering a specified range of services. Although the PACE statute does not specify the states' role in the application approval process, many aspects of implementing PACE in Medicare and Medicaid will necessitate the extensive involvement of the state administering agencies and the state Medicaid agencies. **With regard to applications, CMS believes the states are in the best position to work with potential organizations to develop programs that meet requirements and are integrated into the states' overall long-term care delivery system**. Therefore, CMS requires that applications for PACE organization status be accompanied by an assurance from the state administering agency

J. Pezzuti
Harrisburg, PA, USA
e-mail: jimpezzuti@pezzuticonsultingllc.com

J. Baskins (✉)
Heath Care Consultant, PACE Project Manager, South Carolina Department of Health and Human Services, Columbia, SC, USA

M. K. McNabney (ed.), *Community-Based Integrated Care for Older Adults*, https://doi.org/10.1007/978-3-031-05137-1_7

indicating that it considers the entity to be qualified to be a PACE organization and that the state is willing to enter into a PACE program agreement with the entity. **CMS will not accept applications from entities that have not obtained these assurances**. To enable a state to make such assurances, an entity would have to establish, to the satisfaction of the state, that it is committed to the PACE model of care; there is sufficient funding for program development and facilities; there is adequate demand for PACE services as shown by demographic analysis; and the entity has hired core PACE staff and has developed contracts for referral arrangements and other program services that the site will not furnish directly.

Entities that are interested in developing a PACE program agreement must work collaboratively with their respective state administering agency to give assurance that the state has submitted or plans to submit a state plan amendment to elect PACE as an optional benefit under its State Medicaid Plan and that the state has established additional requirements for PACE organizations.

PACE programs should develop close relationships with their respective state Medicaid programs due to the regulatory and financial requirements involved. Every state is different when it comes to the population it serves, the budget it allocates for health services, and the amount of innovation that is desired in long-term services and support. Therefore, every PACE program must understand the unique needs and requirements of its state. Providers seeking to develop PACE must clearly understand the organizational structure for Medicaid, licensure, and the relationship with the aging network. They must grasp how these different functions impact PACE programs and assure that each stakeholder is part of the conversations to initiate PACE in a given state.

Medicaid and Prospective Providers: Building Support

Incorporating PACE as a service in the state takes committed effort by both Medicaid staff and potential providers that are interested in operating a PACE program. A clear imperative needs to be set forth to successfully navigate the naysayers.

PACE is a prescriptive program that is outlined in the regulations, the PACE manual, and the three-way agreement between the state, CMS, and provider. Additionally, **there are many Technical Assistance Center (TAC) sites that providers can contract with to assist them in building their PACE program and teach them how to operate it**. TACs can also answer many questions posed by the Medicaid agency. However, most states are more than willing to help other states by answering their questions and sharing contracts and specific state issues that do not concern CMS. Developing a PACE Program and running it is almost like following a recipe from a cookbook. Medicaid staff will find PACE to be one of the easiest, if not the easiest, programs to implement in their state. Many systems are already in play as a result of managed care programs within the state Medicaid system that are needed to implement PACE. Adding a new provider type and a few edits to the system usually is not a significant challenge.

Why PACE?

The needs of the elderly vary greatly. There is not one single program, service, or provider that can meet all of the needs of the state's long-term care population. Some individuals simply need daily checks, while other individuals need a great deal of care. This care can take the form of nursing facility (NF) care for those individuals who may not be able to be maintained at home or may be through programs for individuals whose needs can be met in the community and prefer to stay home.

PACE brings to the community a full suite of services an older adult may need to successfully stay at home as long as possible. In addition to having a full range of services, it brings together the staff needed to provide these services to the community. Payrolls are a significant benefit to underserved and economically depressed regions.

No matter what the steps to development are in a state, educating and aligning political leaders are valuable for potential PACE providers to expand awareness of the PACE model of care and how it can positively impact the frail elderly in a community.

State Policy Decisions

State Plan Amendment

A State Medicaid Plan is a contract between a state and the federal government, whereby the state agrees to administer the Medicaid program in accordance with federal law and policy. The State Plan preprint sets forth the scope of the Medicaid program, including groups covered, services furnished, and payment policy. When a state completes a new State Plan preprint page due to changes in its Medicaid program (called a "State Medicaid Plan Amendment"), the preprint page must be approved by CMS in order for the state to receive federal matching funds. Section 1905(a) (26) of the PACE Act, as added by section 4802(a) (1) of the Balanced Budget Act (BBA), provides authority for states to elect PACE as an optional Medicaid benefit. The State Plan electing the optional PACE program must be approved before CMS can approve an application for a PACE organization in that state. CMS has developed a State Plan preprint for PACE.

Administering Agency

Each state must have a state administering agency that is responsible for administering PACE program agreements. The state administering agency closely cooperates with CMS in establishing procedures for entering into, extending, and terminating

PACE program agreements. The state administering agency cooperates with CMS and the PACE organization in the development of participant health status and quality of life outcome measures. The state administering agency cooperates with CMS in conducting oversight reviews of PACE programs and has the authority to terminate a PACE program agreement for a cause.

In many cases, the Medicaid agency contracts with administering agencies, such as departments or agencies that administer various aging programs. It is important that the administering agency clearly understands the Medicaid regulations, the goals of the program, and what role there might be in overseeing the program.

Licensure/Legislation

This can be a difficult area to address. First, a state must address whether the PACE program qualifies under the state's insurance department as an offering that meets its requirement to hold a license from insurance. There are two issues that are typically evaluated to make that determination. *What is being insured?* Insurance licensing is meant to protect the insured member with funds that are available to pay for services received by the member. Since Medicaid and Medicare are the payers, they are the ones at financial risk, not the PACE member. In the event of closure, the member simply reverts to the Medicaid's fee-for-service (FFS) program or their managed care program. The member is never at risk of losing services.

Many state insurance regulations require licensing if the carrier can "subcapitate" their risk-off to a provider. An example would be a managed care organization (MCO), which subcapitates to a hospital regarding types of admissions, thereby shifting its risk to the hospital. States can address this issue in their state-only agreement with the provider (if they chose to implement one in addition to the three-way program agreement) by specifically *not* allowing a PACE provider to subcapitate (subcontract with a provider in a capitated manner). Before including this type of restraint for a PACE program to diversify its business model, the state should consider what other managed care options under Medicare or Medicaid might serve a similar population as PACE and who might wish to subcontract with a PACE program to provide PACE services under Medicare or Medicaid funding. If PACE programs wish to do this, they may need to request a waiver under the BIPA waiver authority to allow the regulatory requirements that anyone enrolled in PACE must be disenrolled from a Medicare or Medicaid managed care plan.

Service Area

One of the unique flexibilities of PACE is that it offers options for states regarding how many PACE providers will serve a particular market. A state can elect to have any PACE provider serve any area they desire, or a state can elect to permit only one PACE provider in a given market area. **PACE serves a market of people aged 55+**

who otherwise qualify for Medicare and/or Medicaid (or who agree to pay privately) and have been determined to be clinically eligible for nursing home care (NFCE) and, at the time of assessment, can be determined to be safely served in the community. Since PACE is very sensitive to market size and is not a mandated program, it is in the interest of both the state and the provider to be certain how many PACE programs a given market area can support. Some states may have more densely populated urban markets where the number of PACE-eligible people is large enough to allow multiple PACE providers. Other areas of a state may be more rural in nature, thereby supporting only one PACE program with enough potential enrollees to assure a sound clinical and fiscal PACE provider.

This is where the importance of a PACE Technical Assistance Center (TAC) comes into play. An interested provider can contract with a TAC, who will review the proposed market areas and determine if the market supports enough potential PACE enrollees (persons who will qualify for PACE) to support a PACE program. At that point, a decision can be made to limit the market to one provider or open it up to multiple providers. Another important consideration is the sizable investment a PACE provider needs to make up front, and the state needs to carefully decide if there is room for more than one provider.

Technical Assistance Center Requirements and Qualifications

Since not all potential providers will have been in the business of managing a program like PACE, the state may want to strongly recommend TAC as part of a contract with a potential provider to help ensure that there are competent advisors assisting the PACE provider to ensure a successful program. The state should consider requiring the potential provider to submit the qualifications of TAC to help ensure the state that the potential provider has procured competent assistance.

Enrollment Limits

In these days of tight budgets, states may be concerned about runaway program budgets and therefore impose enrollment limits. Although it is a state's decision to award a specific number of slots, states are increasingly likely to acknowledge PACE as a managed care model and not arbitrarily limit growth in a full risk model.

Medicaid Rate Setting

PACE programs operate through a three-way partnership, including the provider, the state, and the federal government. While the federal government provides overarching guidance regarding rate setting, PACE Medicaid capitation rates are negotiated between PACE organizations and the states. **Federal regulations require states to set prospective monthly capitation rates consistent with the following criteria: (1) the capitation rate is less than the amount the states would have paid if the participants were not enrolled in PACE programs, (2) the rate accounts for the frailty of the PACE participants, (3) the rate is a fixed amount regardless of changes in the participant's health status, and (4) the rate can be renegotiated on an annual basis.** To ensure that Medicaid rates comply with federal regulations, the Centers for Medicare & Medicaid Services (CMS) reviews the rate-setting approach of each state. The focus of the CMS review is to confirm that Medicaid rates for PACE are no greater than the corresponding upper payment limits (UPLs). Upper payment limits are estimates of the amount the state otherwise would have paid to provide care for individuals similar to those served by the PACE program.

In 2015, CMS issued rate-setting guidance that included expectations on how the state would document and calculate the amount that otherwise would have been paid for a comparable population and expectations for the development and documentation of the PACE rates [3]. States generally use three different approaches to set Medicaid capitation rates for PACE programs; these are listed in Table 7.1. When setting Medicaid payment rates, states also may consider an enrollee's eligibility status, age, and/or geographic location.

The majority of PACE programs currently operating have rates for individuals with Medicaid-only coverage distinct from those who are dually eligible for Medicare and Medicaid coverage [5]. The state Medicaid-only rate tends to be substantially higher than the dual Medicaid rate to compensate for the fact that PACE organizations provide the same services to Medicaid-only participants but do not receive the Medicare portion from the federal government.

Some states calculate distinct PACE payment rates based on age. When rates are based on age, states typically distinguish between enrollees ages 55–64 and those 65 and over.

In states where managed long-term service and support (MLTSS) programs are the dominant delivery model for serving older adults and people with disabilities, FFS data are quickly diminishing.

As FFS data become less available, states are considering approaches other than using a percentage of the UPL to set rates. For example, California, Florida, New

Table 7.1 State approaches to setting medicaid rates for PACE

1. Using a percentage of the Upper Payment Limit (UPL)[a]
2. Using PACE experience to set the monthly PACE capitation rate based on the services provided, cost reports, or a combination of the two in previous time periods trended forward to the current rate period
3. Using Medicaid Long-Term Services and Supports (MLTSS) experience to set the PACE capitation rate based on the actual or expected cost of services provided to a comparable population through managed care plans

[a]Upper Payment Limits = estimates of the amount the state would have otherwise paid to provide care for individuals similar to those served by the PACE program

Jersey, New York, and Wisconsin have begun using alternative approaches for rate setting. The two alternative approaches that states commonly use are setting rates based on PACE cost and utilization experience and setting them based on MLTSS cost and utilization experience. The approach using PACE experience reflects the actual costs incurred by the PACE program, with adjustments to provide a margin for risk reserves to cover higher than expected costs and, in some cases, to account for expected "managed care efficiency" (savings attributable to care coordination). Another approach is based on MLTSS experience, where PACE rates are developed through an actuarial approach using MLTSS cost experience (based on encounter data and MCO financial reports) to estimate utilization rates for services covered by PACE in the comparable population. The total costs are estimated by assigning unit prices to each service or actual health plan payment rates to providers for covered services. In addition, New York and Wisconsin use risk-adjusted models in their rate setting for MLTSS programs, including PACE. Risk adjustment is a statistical method for modifying capitation rates paid to health plans based on the characteristics (e.g., demographics, coverage, acuity, and frailty) of the population they enroll. These characteristics are used to predict the expected costs of providing care to their enrollees. Risk adjustment models have been used for many years by Medicare and Medicaid to adjust rates paid to health plans. Using risk adjustment models for MLTSS programs can account for differences in functional status, a key driver of LTSS costs. Using a risk-adjusted model in developing PACE rates can help reflect the costs of providing care to PACE enrollees based on their characteristics, including frailty.

State Operational Issues

Procurement Process

There are usually two reasons a state is interested in starting up a PACE program, apart from saving money: a provider may have approached it in a market area, or there are market areas that the state believes a PACE program could help provide services, usually economically and service-depressed areas, both rural and urban. It is suggested that the state develops a request for information (RFI) to determine provider interest in developing a PACE program. Responses will come from providers that are already interested in PACE or providers that just started to think about developing a PACE program and their interest was piqued by the state's inquiry.

After a state determines the amount of interest, the state has two choices depending on its procurement rules: (1) develop an RFI or RFP (request for proposal) process or (2) develop provider qualifications and a contract with rates established and then take all comers that qualify. The former is a laborious process, while the latter is very streamlined. The best route depends on the responses from the RFI and how tight and detailed the contract would be.

State Staffing

If the state requires a potential PACE provider to have a TAC (which eliminates a lot of support pressure needed by the potential provider), the state will typically need to commit one-and-a half FTEs, plus system support time, to do the necessary system modifications. It cannot be overstated that PACE is one of the easiest programs for Medicaid to offer to one of its most vulnerable populations. Other state staff who have gone through implementation are usually quite willing to share contracts, rate-setting ideas, policies, and procedures. A state looking to implement PACE can reach out to other states for help in creating a strategy to more likely have successful implementation.

Separate Medicaid Agreement

As mentioned earlier, there is a three-way agreement between CMS, the state, and the provider. CMS is primarily interested in having the agreement address their requirements. States that have additional reporting requirements (state-specific issues) must have a separate contract with the provider. Usually, this agreement addresses specific state-required reports, processes, or other issues not of interest to CMS. Examples of these contracts can be obtained from other states as a template to think through issues that are not addressed by the three-way agreement.

Enrollment Agreement 42 CFR § 460.154 (CFR—Code of Federal Regulations)

The minimum requirements for an enrollment agreement are available in the CFR. **The enrollment agreement is very clear about the PACE provider network, such as hospital systems, that is used and that the provider agreement should be available to the member in the language that the member and their support understand**. There are many examples of enrollment agreements that are available to states interested in implementing PACE. Any financial obligations of the member, such as patient-pay obligations by the member, must be delineated.

The state should ensure that the enrollment agreement for persons whose primary language is not English must be reviewed and approved by persons who are culturally competent and who understand subtleties that can make a big difference in interpretation. A person who speaks another language is not necessarily culturally competent. A clear, concise enrollment agreement can smoothen the way for a productive relationship between the PACE provider and the member. CMS has a very regimented process for the revirew of marketing materials for PACE Programs This includes the review of PACE Participant enrollment agreements.

Process for Enrollment

The state needs to be clear about how to enroll a member into PACE, independent of meeting CMS regulatory requirements. What agency or organization determines "nursing facility clinically eligible" (NFCE)? Where does one go to determine their financial eligibility? Who advises the potential member of all options prior to deciding to enroll in any program?

These are stopping points that states already have in play for other programs. States are processing hundreds of financial applications for numerous programs every day. PACE is different in that the PACE provider must perform an initial assessment to decide at the time of their assessment that an applicant can be safely served in the community. Then the NFCE determination is made by the appropriate agent and forwarded for processing to determine financial eligibility. States may delegate the assessment process to PACE programs to confirm nursing home eligibility, but the final approval is typically retained by the state to verify this aspect of PACE eligibility. This process is required, whether or not a potential PACE enrollee is Medicaid eligible.

Reporting Requirements

Financial

While CMS has no standardized PACE financial formats, states may wish to require standardized cost reports from their PACE providers with the accompanying balance sheet. First, it can help inform the state about rate setting, in addition to the process for determining positive net worth. Reviewing cost centers as to where money is being spent is less important than where money is not being spent. Using cost reports as part of an overall quality assurance process makes the cost report more useful than looking for net positive worth.

CMS requires the submission of quarterly financial reports *during the first 3 years of operations*, and the financials are then audited 180 days after the close of each fiscal year *for all PACE programs*. States have access to this information in the Health Plan Management System (HPMS) but can also have their own reporting requirements. The ongoing monitoring of fiscal solvency and risk reserve typically falls on the state. Many states have established fiscal solvency requirements that build upon CMS regulatory requirements to ensure the fiscal soundness of a PACE Program.

Readiness Reviews

The purpose of this review is to determine the organization's readiness to administer the PACE program and enroll participants. The State Readiness Review must determine if the PACE program applicant (1) meets the requirements stipulated in the PACE regulation, (2) has developed policies and procedures consistent with the PACE regulation, and (3) has established the contracts necessary to provide all-inclusive, quality care to its participants. The Readiness Review and Compliance Report can be downloaded to assist state and potential providers in deciding whether to move forward with establishing a PACE program. A provider will have a considerable outlay in capital prior to enrolling its first member. State Readiness Reviews are conducted as part of the PACE application process and typically occur after the PACE application has completed the initial review by CMS.

Reporting

The “PACE Quality Monitoring & Reporting Guidance” is available on the CMS website for review by states and provider organizations (POs) considering implementing a PACE program. It is very important that POs build their systems to capture this information upfront. There are companies that have developed software designed to capture this information and other data useful for operating an effective PACE organization. States are free to add their own requirements to capture information unique to their requirements and would be advised to talk with other states to get their comments on the usefulness of the proposed data elements.

For states that do not have the capacity to accept encounter data and/or quality data from PACE programs, the National PACE Association has developed and refined, over time, data collected by members as part of their DataPACE initiative. PACE programs may grant states access to this information, which can benchmark both quality and encounter reporting metrics nationally.

Federal Medicaid managed care regulations require states to collect encounters from Medicaid managed care plans and submit them to CMS. The federal requirement is long-standing, but poor compliance in many states led CMS to add a strong enforcement measure in the Final Medicaid Managed Care Rule of 2016, making the receipt of federal matching funds for payments made to managed care plans conditional on the submission of validated, complete, and timely enrollee encounter data. Federal compliance aside, states use encounter data to monitor quality and utilization, calculate and validate rates, and conduct evaluation and research studies. The federal PACE rule does not mandate encounter reporting, but a handful of states have begun requiring PACE organizations to submit them. State officials report that PACE encounters are beneficial for comparing PACE with other service delivery models, developing risk-adjustment methods, and setting rates. However, the unique nature of the PACE model creates several challenges for encounter reporting.

PACE organizations are essentially hybrids of managed care plans and provider organizations. They receive capitated Medicaid and Medicare payments and pay network providers like plans, and they also employ clinical and ancillary staff and provide intensive services directly in centers, alternative care sites, and participant's homes. While at a center, a participant receives several encounters a day from multiple staff and multiple encounters from a single staff person. On the way to the center, participants encounter van drivers and attendants. A participant's interdisciplinary team (IDT) meeting is typically an in-person meeting comprised of several clinical and nonclinical staff. These attributes are central to the PACE model, yet many of them are not captured easily through the standard 837 encounter format.

If states are considering requiring encounter reporting, those conversations should happen as soon in the PACE development process as possible to allow the PACE program not only to collect the data but also to have systems at the state level that can receive the information. Clearly understanding the usage of the data is important.

Ongoing Monitoring

Ongoing monitoring is both state and CMS requirements. Beginning in 2017, CMS restructured its auditing process to focus on compliance with CMS regulations, and the role of the states became limited in the audit process. Subsequently, many states have developed their own approach to ongoing monitoring and oversight. How states have implemented this process varies dramatically from state to state and depends heavily on the resources at the state level as to how robust the processes are or are not.

The Programs of All-Inclusive Care for the Elderly (PACE) Audit Overview Medicare Parts C and D Oversight and Enforcement Group Division of Analysis, Policy, and Strategy is available for download. PACE audit fieldwork is usually conducted over a period of 2 weeks. Key milestones (described in the audit overview document) include the following:

1. ***Entrance conference***—audit fieldwork begins with an entrance conference held on the morning of the first day of fieldwork. The audit leader conducts the meeting, reviews the schedule, and discusses expectations for the audit. The PACE organization will also have an opportunity to make a presentation about its organization.
2. ***Audit fieldwork week 1***—the first week of the audit includes a review of the service delivery, appeals, and grievance element and may include a review of additional elements, when possible, via a desk review or webinar (this may also include remote access to the PACE organization's medical records).
3. ***Audit fieldwork week 2***—the second week of audit fieldwork includes an in-person audit conducted at one or more PACE centers (or alternative care settings). The location(s) of the in-person audit will be determined by CMS. The second week will include a review of all elements not conducted during the first week of audit fieldwork, in-person participant observations, and, when necessary, a review of sample cases or medical records for elements started, but not

completed, during the first week of audit fieldwork. At the beginning of the second week, the PACE organization must submit the information identified in the Onsite Observation Participant List.

Complaints and Grievances

A grievance is defined as a complaint, either written or oral, expressing dissatisfaction with the service delivery or the quality of care furnished. The PACE organization must have a formal written process to evaluate and resolve grievances, whether medical or nonmedical in nature, by PACE participants, their family members, or representatives. All personnel (employees and contractors) who have contact with participants should be aware of and understand the basic procedures for receiving and documenting grievances in order to initiate the appropriate process for resolving participant concerns**. All participants must be informed of the grievance process in writing upon enrollment into the PACE program and at least annually thereafter**.

It is extremely important for PACE staff to be aware that any expression by a member needs to be properly documented and that a written resolution be provided to a member.

Appeals

An appeal is defined as a participant's action taken against a PACE organization's noncoverage or nonpayment of service, including denials, reductions, or termination of services. The PACE organization must have a formal, written appeal process in place, including time frames for responding to the noncoverage or nonpayment of a service. **All participants must be provided written information regarding the appeal process upon enrollment and at least annually thereafter and whenever the IDT denies a request for services or payment**. It is expected that each PACE organization has a template prepared to assist the participant in filing an appeal, with a written notification to acknowledge that a participant has appealed within the required time frame, with additional information on the process, and with a notice of action providing the appeal outcome as well as information on the next level of appeal. The information on appeal proceedings will be maintained, aggregated, and analyzed by the organization. This process will be utilized as a part of the organization's internal quality program. By analyzing the filed appeals, there may be an opportunity to improve the process, which could lead to improved quality of care for the participants.

For the "dual eligible" population, a member can choose either Medicare's or Medicaid's appeal process.

Disenrollment and Involuntary Disenrollment

A member can voluntarily disenroll from PACE at any time without reason, although the most common reason is moving out of the service area.

Although it is unusual, a member may be involuntarily disenrolled (42 CFR§ 460.164.) A participant may be involuntarily disenrolled for any of the following reasons:

1. The participant, after a 30-day grace period, fails to pay or make satisfactory arrangements to pay any premium due to the PACE organization.
2. The participant, after a 30-day grace period, fails to pay or make satisfactory arrangements to pay any applicable Medicaid spend-down liability or any amount due under the posteligibility treatment of income process.
3. The participant or the participant's caregiver engages in disruptive or threatening behavior.
4. The participant moves out of the PACE program service area or is out of the service area for more than 30 consecutive days, unless the PACE organization agrees to a longer absence due to extenuating circumstances.
5. The participant is determined to no longer meet the state Medicaid nursing facility level of care requirements and is not deemed eligible.
6. The PACE program agreement with CMS and the state administering agency is not renewed or is terminated.
7. The PACE organization is unable to offer health care services due to the loss of state licenses or contracts with outside providers.

Eligibility

To qualify for PACE, a person must be aged 55 or over, live in a PACE service area, and be certified by the state to need a nursing home level care and at the point of enrollment can be safely cared for in the community. The criteria to define the ability to be safely cared for in the community are developed by each state and are included in the three-way program agreement. Additionally, an applicant must meet financial requirements. For private pay applicants with or without Medicare, they must still be certified by the state to need a nursing home level care.

Enrollment

The PACE-eligible applicant/prospective enrollee (or legal representative) must agree to several enrollment conditions, including but not limited to having the **PACE organization and its provider network as the sole provider**

of services, giving **signed consent for the PACE organization to obtain medical and financial information to verify eligibility**, and **agreeing to any applicable monthly premiums or Medicaid spend-down obligations**. If the prospective PACE enrollee meets the eligibility requirements and signs the PACE enrollment agreement, the effective date of enrollment in the PACE program is on the first day of the calendar month following the date the PACE organization receives the participant's signed enrollment agreement. The PACE organization must submit a timely and accurate enrollment transaction to complete the enrollment in CMS systems. Detailed requirements are listed in the PACE enrollment regulations.

Prospective states looking to implement PACE would be advised to secure examples of different enrollment agreements from other states and standardize the enrollment language for use by POs in their state, leaving a particular section for the PO to deal **with who they are, their network, and other information unique to their organization and region**.

Three-Way Program Agreement

CMS requires that each PACE organization have an agreement with CMS and the state administering agency for the operation of a PACE program by the organization under Medicare and Medicaid. This three-party agreement must be signed by an authorized official of the organization, as well as by an authorized CMS official and an authorized state official.

The content and terms of the PACE program agreement are defined in CFR (§ 460.32) in § 460.32(a).

Stakeholder Education, Communication, and Buy-in

Internal

The Medicaid agency or its designee must decide where the PACE program management will "reside" within its agency. Typically, PACE has resided in the bureau/division that deals with its long-term care programs and waivers. As PACE at the state level becomes more aligned with the state's managed long-term care strategy, PACE may well reside in this area of Medicaid than home and community-based services, which identify PACE as more of an extension of their waivered services than a fully capitated managed care model.

Staff who are assigned in these areas need to become familiar with PACE, how it operates, and the regulatory framework. This is best accomplished by first going to a state that has a PACE program, then touring its PACE site, and then asking questions of the provider and the state staff in order to get an overall feel of how PACE programs operate from a state perspective. As PACE has grown, so has the knowledge and expertise of states that provide oversight to PACE programs. These states are very collaborative and are willing to share with developing states their knowledge and expertise.

Spending time on the National PACE Association website will also be informative. After the staff is generally informed about PACE, it can produce salient talking points to keep everyone on the same page. These talking points will be needed to gain support from other state agencies and the overall stakeholder group.

Affected Offices

Offices within the Medicaid agency and potentially those outside Medicaid (if their areas of responsibility impact aspects of PACE operations) will need to be briefed, and specific talking points need to be drafted to address their unique concerns. Those individuals responsible for data systems may need coaching through implementation. They will need to add a provider code for PACE providers and interface the payment system with the system that captures financial and program eligibility. Typically, modern system designs allow this process to happen without an excessive amount of time compared to the systems of old. Again, it is recommended to work with other states that have implemented PACE.

Authority

Departments like Health and Insurance will need to determine their direct involvement in implementing PACE. These two departments are usually involved with health insurers, such as MCOs, by licensing them to operate within their state and enacting various regulations that apply to them.

Fortunately, CMS has determined that PACE is not a Medicare Advantage plan, so the only issue at hand is whether PACE meets the state's requirement as a product that meets the state definition of an insurer. If so, it needs to be a *licensed* insurer. Most states have determined that this is not the case with PACE for three reasons: the member has no money at risk, the PO provides nearly all of the services, and the PO is prohibited from shifting risk to another provider.

Licensing agencies—some states require some form of licensing, while other states do not. Usually, if there is a license, it only applies to the Adult Day Center, which addresses the physical space of a PACE Center. Before deciding on the need for licensure, it is advised to carefully review the PACE regulations; the three-way

CMS, state, and PO agreement; and the various local health and building code regulations to determine if there is an actual need for an additional state license.

The other most prominent license applied to PACE is home health, which varies state by state and is dependent on how the licensing requirements for home care are worded.

Whatever applies, it is important to determine why they are necessary. State-specific licensing criteria when applied to PACE can often conflict with CMS PACE regulations and require a duplication of effort with little to no added value.

Legislators

Depending on the state, some type of program revision statement is used to authorize the allotment of money for the PACE program or, at least, its addition as a program covered by the current long-term care program funding. Arguably, PACE will shift money from a provider type/line item, such as a nursing facility payment, to a less expensive PACE line item. Very little new money is needed over and above the state's current growth curve. Additionally, legislators are always interested in job growth in their districts that are economically depressed zones, such as rural areas. PACE brings well-paying jobs to areas where services are scarce, in addition to being a less expensive program regardless of where it occurs within the state.

External

Nursing Home Industry

This group is usually the most impacted by a PACE program in terms of overall bed occupancy. PACE's utilization of beds ranges typically from 8% to 12% of their members occupying NF beds, either temporarily or through permanent placement. Additionally, hospital use by PACE members generally declines. For states that are addressing the rebalancing of long-term care programs from institutional to home and community-based services, PACE has an important role in helping states achieve this. This is typically seen as a high likelihood of savings for the state.

Home Care

Home care providers could be impacted by PACE, depending on the PACE program contracting with them, to provide home-based services when members are not in the center. Many POs prefer to contract with home health agencies and home care providers to avoid additional licensing requirements.

Advocacy Organizations

It is important that time is spent with advocacy agencies. Discussions need to be open and transparent to avoid a possible concern about a capitated program. PACE is a uniquely different program in that it cannot shift itself out of risk. If PACE does not provide the best possible care for its members, the PO will pay the higher price of emergency room (ER) visits and preventable hospitalizations. Once time is spent educating advocates, they usually become supporters.

Role of Community/Advisory Committees

A PACE organization is required to develop a committee(s) with community input to (1) evaluate data collected pertaining to quality outcome measures, (2) address the implementation of and results from the Quality Improvement Program plan, and (3) provide input related to ethical decision-making, including end-of-life issues and the implementation of the Patient Self-Determination Act. Through this committee(s), the PACE organization will be able to receive guidance regarding its QI program and the ethical issues faced by PACE organizations and by regulations.

There are various committees that oversee these requirements. It is imperative that they are active, engaged, and have appropriate community members on their boards. The regulations outline these committees and responsibilities.

Interaction with Medicare + Choice

Although the PACE program has certain fundamental similarities to Medicare Advantage and managed care organizations, PACE is not a Medicare Advantage plan. PACE is similar to some Medicare Advantage options in these ways: it is capitated, it is risk-based, it provides managed care, and it is an elective option. However, PACE differs significantly from the Medicare Advantage plan in other ways, such as the following: it is not available nationwide (only in a limited number of sites), it includes statutory waivers that expand the scope of Medicare-covered services, it is not available to all beneficiaries (only to a defined subset of frail elderly), and it is a joint Medicare/Medicaid program.

In turn, PACE is a form of Medicaid managed care, but it also does not comply with many of the regulatory requirements that apply to managed care options offered to Medicaid beneficiaries. As more states are developing strategies to align Medicare and Medicaid funding and managed care around the needs of a dual-eligible population, they should closely examine the strategic differences that apply to each. In addition, they should be aware of decisions that are made for Medicaid managed care, especially managed long-term support services and how they can negatively impact PACE programs.

Things to Consider

1. Lengthy enrollment process – PACE programs can have a prolonged enrollment process that requires assessments to verify the clinical eligibility for enrollment into the program. This can be a time-consuming process that prevents PACE from immediately enrolling an individual who needs the services of the program but delays that actual enrollment to the first day of the next calendar month. Waiver services can immediately enroll someone, which results in an individual receiving some services but not the comprehensive service delivery system that PACE offers.
2. Autoenrollment verses complicated enrollment process for PACE—MLTSS plans can participate in a state's autoenrollment process. Due to the eligibility requirements of PACE programs serving a frail elderly population, they are not able to utilize this autoenrollment process. PACE programs typically have to find potential enrollees and bring them to the door of an enrollment broker, who then processes the applicant as an enrollee in PACE. This puts PACE at an unfair disadvantage in growing their census.
3. PACE rate setting – as previously discussed, PACE programs are required by statute not to cost no more than a comparable population. MLTSS programs do not have these constraints and may in some cases actually receive rates higher than PACE while not providing the same individualized care that PACE does.
4. Limits on PACE enrollment – many states apply slot limits to PACE enrollment, which not only limits program growth but also does not allow them to compete with managed care options that have no limit on growth and enrollment.
5. Option counseling – option counseling is offered by many states in some fashion often through their respective Departments of Aging Services. Secret shopper approaches to option counseling revealed that they have little to no knowledge of PACE and are unsure how to guide a caller in the direction of a PACE program that could better suit their needs.

The National PACE Association has assimilated resources available to states to help address some of these concerns as states are developing and implementing their managed long-term care strategies.

Summary

All PACE programs must collaborate with the state Medicaid program on aspects of development, start-up, operation, and regulatory compliance. There must be a full commitment at the state level for this form of community-based integrated care to be successful. As all states move toward "rebalancing" how Medicaid dollars are expended in long-term care, community-based alternatives to nursing home care will become increasingly prominent as a provider of care. Technical assistance centers (TACs) are valuable to PACE programs as they develop and grow, providing detailed information that is crucial to success. There are many aspects that require state-specific oversight, which include regulations and financing.

Suggested Reading

1. Department of Health And Human Services, Centers for Medicare & Medicaid Services, 42 CFR Parts 423 and 460, [CMS–4168–F], RIN 0938–AR60, Medicare and Medicaid Programs; Programs of All-Inclusive Care for the Elderly (PACE).
2. Gross DL, Temkin-Greener H, Kunitz S, Mukamel DB. The growing pains of integrated health care for the elderly: lessons from the expansion of PACE. Milbank Q. 2004;82:257–82.
3. Mui AC. The Program of All-Inclusive Care for the Elderly (PACE): an innovative long-term care model in the United States. J Aging Soc Policy. 2001;13:53–67.

Chapter 8
Medication Management and Part D Coverage in PACE

Catherine Knuth, Richard Mueller, Kathryn Dorward King, and Ashley Souza

What Is Medicare Part D?

The 2006 Medicare Modernization Act (MMA) established the Medicare Part D program to provide outpatient prescription drug coverage to older adults and people with disabilities who are eligible for Medicare. Part D coverage is funded by federal Medicare dollars and can be provided via a Medicare Advantage plan with drug coverage (MA-PD) or a stand-alone Prescription Drug Plan (PDP). An MA-PD plan covers medical services as well as prescription drug services, whereas a PDP adds prescription drug coverage to original Medicare or another plan that covers Medicare-funded medical services but not prescription drugs.

Medicare beneficiaries with limited income and assets are eligible for assistance with Part D plan premiums and cost sharing through the Part D Low-Income Subsidy (LIS) program. Currently, most PACE participants are low-income dual eligibles (eligible for both federal Medicare and state Medicaid benefits). Very few people who are not eligible for Medicaid (i.e., Medicare-only participants) enroll in PACE because they would have to pay a significant monthly premium to cover the

C. Knuth (✉)
Milliman, Brookfield, WI, USA
e-mail: catherine.knuth@milliman.com

R. Mueller
Mequon, WI, USA
e-mail: rjmueller@wi.rr.com

K. D. King
Rochester, NY, USA
e-mail: kathryn.dorward@rochesterregional.org

A. Souza
Neighborhood PACE, East Boston, MA, USA
e-mail: souzaa@ebnhc.org

M. K. McNabney (ed.), *Community-Based Integrated Care for Older Adults*,
https://doi.org/10.1007/978-3-031-05137-1_8

amount the state Medicaid program pays for a dual-eligible participant, plus a portion of the Part D premium, as described later in this chapter.

The Medicare Part D program is administered by the Centers for Medicare & Medicaid Services (CMS) within the US Department of Health and Human Services (HHS). PACE organizations are considered "Part D sponsors" and provide outpatient prescription drugs to their participants via the Part D program. The remainder of this chapter will describe Part D as it relates to PACE, including the Part D benefit, how PACE organizations are paid for Part D services, required Part D experience reporting, the Part D payment reconciliation process, and Part D compliance requirements.

Part D Benefits

Each year, CMS defines the standard Part D benefit, and Part D sponsors are required to provide prescription drug benefits that are actuarially equivalent to or richer than the standard Part D benefit. Table 8.1 summarizes the 2022 standard low-income Part D benefit for dual-eligible participants.

PACE organizations are required to provide 100% coverage of prescription drugs to their participants, but the parameters of the standard Part D benefit impact how CMS reimburses PACE organizations for Part D, as described later in this chapter.

Part D Payments

PACE organizations receive a monthly Part D premium payment from the Centers for Medicare & Medicaid Services (CMS) equal to the premium amount CMS calculates for each PACE participant. Each participant's premium reflects the expected cost for the PACE organization to provide Medicare Part D covered prescription drugs to enrolled participants.

Table 8.1 Standard low-income Part D benefit for dual-eligible beneficiaries calendar year 2022

Corridor name	Participant responsibility
Deductible	100% of the first $480 in annual Part D drug costs
Initial Coverage Limit	25% of the next $3,950 (up to $4,430) in annual Part D drug costs
Coverage Gap [a]	100% of the next $5,582.50 (up to $10,012.50) in annual Part D drug costs
Catastrophic Limit	Greater than $3.95/$9.85 per generic/brand script or 5% over $10,012.50 in annual Part D drug costs

(This table was created by the authors with information publicly available from CMS.)
[a]The standard member coinsurance for non-dual eligibles is 25% (generic)/95% (brand) of the next $5,582.50

Table 8.2 Part D payment responsibility based on participant type

Subsidy	Dual eligible	Medicare only
Basic Premium	CMS	Participant
Direct Subsidy	CMS	CMS
Reinsurance Subsidy	CMS	N/A
Low-Income Cost-Sharing Subsidy	CMS	N/A
PACE Subsidy	CMS	N/A
Supplemental Premium	N/A	Participant

(This table was created by the authors with information publicly available from CMS.)

As summarized in Table 8.2 below, dual-eligible participants do not pay a premium for Part D coverage, but Medicare-only participants must pay a portion of the expected cost via a monthly premium.

The sum of the basic premium and direct subsidy is often referred to as the "Part D Bid" and is the per member per month (PMPM) amount needed to cover the Part D sponsor's portion of the standard Part D benefit, including the covered Part D drug cost, non-benefit (administrative) expenses, and a gain/loss (i.e., profit) margin. The covered Part D drug cost includes the drug ingredient costs, dispensing fees, sales tax, and administration fees for vaccines not covered under the Medicare Part B benefit. The non-benefit expense represents the expected administrative cost of providing the Part D benefit and includes the following types of expenses:

- Direct administration expenses —expenses directly attributable to Medicare Part D.
- Sales and marketing expenses—a portion of the costs attributable to marketing the PACE organization to eligible participants.
- Indirect administration expenses—a portion of overhead expenses indirectly attributable to Medicare Part D.

For dual-eligible participants, CMS also pays the following subsidies which, combined with the basic premium and direct subsidy, are intended to cover 100% of the revenue needed to provide Part D benefits:

- **Reinsurance Subsidy**—CMS provides reinsurance coverage equal to 80% of all dual-eligible participants' costs over the Medicare Part D catastrophic limit.
- **Low Income Cost Sharing (LICS) Subsidy–** since PACE organizations are not allowed to collect cost sharing (i.e., deductibles, copays, and coinsurance) from participants, CMS pays most of the standard Part D cost sharing that would have been paid by the participant through the Low Income Cost Sharing Subsidy. CMS pays the remainder of the participant's cost sharing through the PACE Subsidy.
- **PACE Subsidy—**since noninstitutionalized dual eligibles must pay a $1.35 generic/$4.00 brand copayment under Part D, which a PACE program is prohibited from collecting, CMS pays PACE organizations an additional PACE Subsidy to cover this cost.

Unlike dual-eligible participants, Medicare-only participants must pay the difference between the 100% PACE benefit and the standard Part D benefit. The Medicare-only participant's premium (i.e., the private pay premium) consists of a standard Part D premium (the Basic Premium) and a Supplemental Premium. The Supplemental Premium covers all of the standard member cost sharing the PACE organization is prohibited from collecting, plus the catastrophic reinsurance the government will not pay due to the 100% benefit.

Part D Risk Adjustment

The Part D bid payment (i.e., the sum of Basic Premium and Direct Subsidy) is different for each participant because CMS adjusts these payments to reflect each participant's Part D risk score. The Reinsurance Subsidy, LICS Subsidy, and PACE Subsidy amounts are not risk adjusted (i.e., they are the same for all participants).

CMS calculates a relative risk score for each Part D beneficiary using its RxHCC Part D risk score model. The objective of the RxHCC model is to use medical diagnosis and other information (such as age, gender, and Medicaid eligibility) to predict each participant's future Part D drug costs. The RxHCC model maps individual diagnoses to disease groups, called Hierarchical Condition Categories (HCCs), each of which has a point value assigned to it. CMS imposes hierarchies among related condition categories so that a person is only coded for the most severe manifestation among related diseases.

CMS uses diagnoses from one year to predict costs in the following year and updates risk scores at least twice in each payment/calendar year:

- CMS calculates each participant's initial Part D risk score using diagnosis data from July 1 of the calendar year 2 years prior to the payment year through June 30 of the calendar year 1 year prior to the payment year (e.g., July 1, 2020 through June 30, 2021 dates of service for the initial 2022 risk scores/payments).
- CMS calculates each participant's mid-year risk score using diagnoses from the prior calendar year (e.g., January 1, 2021 through December 31, 2021 dates of service for the mid-year 2022 risk scores payments). CMS applies the mid-year risk score updates retroactively to the payments made in prior months of the calendar year (e.g., 2022).
- CMS calculates each participant's final risk score after the end of the calendar year and applies the final risk score updates retroactively to the prior payments made for the calendar year. The final risk scores use diagnoses from the same dates of service as the mid-year risk scores but include additional diagnosis information that was not available at the time CMS calculated the mid-year risk scores.

PACE organizations submit diagnoses to CMS through the Risk Adjustment Processing System (RAPS) and the Encounter Data System (EDS). PACE organizations are only required to submit encounters for services provided for which they collect a claim form, and CMS combines the diagnoses from the two sources to determine risk scores. **It is critical for PACE organizations to document and capture all appropriate diagnosis codes in their RAPS and EDS files to make sure they are paid appropriately for the risks enrolled**.

CMS uses the same medical diagnosis data to calculate two separate risk scores for each participant—one that predicts medical costs and is used to determine the PACE organization's Medicare Part A and B payments and one that predicts drug costs and is used to determine Part D payments. The risk score for participants with no diagnosis data is based on age and gender, Medicaid eligibility, and originally disabled status only. Risk scores for new PACE participants are based on diagnosis data submitted to CMS by the participant's prior plan (if such data exist).

Part D Experience Reporting

CMS requires Part D sponsors to report their prescription drug event (PDE) experience on a script-level basis in a prescribed format, including the following types of information:

- General (e.g., submitter ID, contract number, date of service, paid date, etc.)
- Demographic (e.g., Medicare Beneficiary Identifier, date of birth, gender, etc.)
- Provider (e.g., service provider ID, prescriber ID, pharmacy service type, etc.)
- Prescription (e.g., National Drug Code (NDC), quantity dispensed, ingredient cost, dispensing fee, etc.)

CMS expects the PDE to be submitted within 30 days of the date the drug was dispensed. After a PACE organization submits a file of PDE records, CMS provides a return file with a code appended to the end of each record indicating whether the record was accepted or rejected. **CMS expects rejected records to be corrected and resubmitted within 90 days of the date of the return file**.

CMS also requires Part D sponsors to report all drug cost adjustments that occur after the point of sale. CMS refers to such adjustments as "direct and indirect remuneration" or "DIR" because the adjustments decrease the costs incurred by the Part D sponsor, either directly or indirectly. Manufacturer rebates are the most common form of DIR reported by PACE organizations, but DIR may also include pharmacy prompt pay discounts, chargebacks, cash discounts, free goods contingent on a purchase agreement, up-front payments, coupons, goods in kind, free or reduced-price services, grants, legal judgment amounts, settlement amounts from lawsuits or other legal action, and other price concessions or similar benefits.

DIR may be paid by any source (manufacturers, pharmacies, enrollees, etc.) and may be received by the PACE organization or by a contracted third party, such as the PACE organization's pharmacy benefits manager (PBM) or pharmacy. **Any DIR received on behalf of the PACE organization, whether paid to the PACE organization or retained by a contracted third party, must be reported as DIR**.

PACE organizations must submit DIR reports to CMS annually—typically by June 30 of the following year—and are required to report summarized DIR for dual eligibles separate from Medicare-only participants, as well as DIR by NDC.

Part D Payment Reconciliation

The Part D premium payments a PACE organization receives from CMS throughout the year are estimates of the PACE organization's cost to provide the Part D benefit. Each year, CMS requires PACE organizations to calculate the expected cost to provide Medicare Part D covered prescription drugs to enrolled participants and to submit these estimates to CMS as part of the Medicare Part D bid process. PACE organizations submit two bids to CMS: one for dual-eligible participants and one for Medicare-only participants. The annual bid process follows guidelines and forms provided by CMS, and all bids must be certified by a qualified actuary.

Approximately 9 months after the end of the calendar year, CMS compares the drug cost portion of the Part D premium paid to each PACE organization during the year with the PACE organization's actual Part D drug costs (as reported in the PDE and DIR files) and performs a payment reconciliation. **If the premium payments were higher than the PACE organization's actual costs, CMS may require the PACE organization to pay them back**. Conversely, if the premium payments were lower than the PACE organization's actual costs, CMS may owe the PACE organization additional payments. The non-benefit expense portion of the Part D premium payments is not subject to year-end reconciliation, although PACE organizations are required to report their non-benefit expenses to CMS in the bid forms for subsequent years.

The final payment reconciliation amount is the sum of three separate calculations: a risk-sharing reconciliation, a reinsurance subsidy reconciliation, and a low-income cost-sharing subsidy reconciliation. Table 8.3 displays the components of Part D premium payments and how CMS reconciles each component.

The Reinsurance Subsidy reconciliation compares the total Reinsurance Subsidy payments received to the portion of the actual cost experience covered by this subsidy. The difference between the payments and the actual costs is the amount owed

Table 8.3 Part D payment reconciliation calculations

Part D payment	Payment reconciliation approach
Basic Premium	Risk sharing
Direct Subsidy	Risk sharing
Reinsurance Subsidy	Payments—Actual costs = amount owed to (from) CMS
Low Income Cost Sharing Subsidy	Payments—Actual costs = amount owed to (from) CMS
PACE Subsidy	Risk sharing

(This table was created by the authors with information publicly available from CMS.)

to or from CMS. Because this subsidy does not apply to Medicare-only participants, CMS does this reconciliation for dual eligibles only.

Similarly, the Low Income Cost Sharing Subisyd reconciliation compares the total Low Income Cost Sharing Subsidy payments received to the portion of the actual cost experience covered by this subsidy. The difference between the payments and the actual costs is the amount owed to or from CMS. Because this subsidy does not apply to Medicare-only participants, CMS does this reconciliation for dual eligibles only.

The risk-sharing calculation compares the standard Part D drug cost portion of the premium payments (i.e., the sum of the Basic Premium and Direct Subsidy payments, adjusted to remove non-benefit expense and gain/(loss), plus the PACE Subsidy) to the portion of the actual Part D cost experience allocated to the standard Part D benefit. **The difference between the payments received and the actual costs incurred is then subject to a risk-sharing formula to determine the amount owed to or from CMS**. Table 8.4 summarizes the risk corridor ratios and risk-sharing reconciliation payments.

In general, the lower the ratio of actual costs to payments received, the more the PACE organization pays to CMS to reimburse a portion of the excess premium payments received during the calendar year. Conversely, the higher the ratio of actual costs to payments received, the more CMS pays to the PACE organization to make up for a portion of the inadequacy of premium payments received during the calendar year. No adjustments occur if the ratio is between 95% and 105%.

PACE organizationsshould monitor their Part D premium payments and actual drug costs throughout the year to determine whether they should establish and maintain a financial reserve or an account receivable and avoid surprises at year-end regarding the direction and size of the reconciliation calculation.

Table 8.4 Part D payment reconciliation risk-sharing calculations

Ratio of actual costs to payments received	Risk-sharing payment calculation
Ratio < 90%	PACE organization pays CMS 50% of 5% of the payments received, plus 80% of the difference between 90% of the payments received and the actual costs; PACE organization retains the remainder
90% < ratio < 95%	PACE organization pays CMS 50% of the difference between 95% of the payments received and the actual costs; PACE organization retains the remainder
95% < ratio < 105%	No adjustment
105% < ratio < 110%	CMS pays PACE organization 50% of the difference between the actual costs and 105% of the payments received; PACE organization is responsible for the remainder
Ratio > 110%	CMS pays PACE organization 50% of 5% of the payments received, plus 80% of the difference between the actual costs and 110% of the payments received; PACE organization is responsible for the remainder

(This table was created by the authors with information publicly available from CMS.)

Part D Compliance

CMS requires each Part D sponsor to implement an effective compliance program to prevent, detect, and correct fraud, waste, and abuse (FWA), as well as determine whether there is any Medicare program noncompliance. Chapter 9 of the CMS Prescription Drug Benefit Manual[1] outlines the Medicare compliance requirements, the key elements of which are as follows:

1. Written policies, procedures, and standards of conduct.
2. Compliance officer, compliance committee, and high-level oversight.
3. Training and education.
4. Lines of communication.
5. Disciplinary standards.
6. Routine monitoring, auditing, and identification of compliance risks.
7. Procedures and systems for prompt response to compliance issues.

PACE organizations are only required to comply with elements 6 and 7, but CMS strongly encourages PACE organizations to comply with the other elements as well.

A PACE organization's PDE data is a valuable source of information for detecting the potential for FWA, and CMS expects PACE organizations to perform claim reviews to help ensure that CMS is not overpaying or underpaying for prescription drugs. In addition to auditing drug payments against the pricing terms in the pharmacy contract(s), PACE organizations can also analyze their PDE data for the following reasons:

- Benchmark their utilization and costs against baseline PACE data.
- Perform physician, patient, and pharmacy profiling.
- Detect billing, dispensing, and pricing anomalies.
- Identify Part D and non-Part D coverage errors.
- Evaluate and minimize early refills.
- Analyze rejected claims.

In addition to being responsible for their own actions, CMS also holds Part D sponsors responsible for the actions of their first tier, downstream, and related entities (FDRs)—any organization with whom a sponsor contracts to provide administrative or health care services to its participants. The following exhibit (Fig. 8.1) displays the illustration of FDRs from Chap. 9 of CMS' Prescription Drug Benefit Manual.

Part D sponsors may not delegate compliance program administrative functions (e.g., compliance officer, compliance committee, compliance reporting to senior management, etc.) to entities other than its parent organization or corporate

[1] https://www.cms.gov/Medicare/Prescription-Drug-Coverage/PrescriptionDrugCovContra/Downloads/Chapter9.pdf

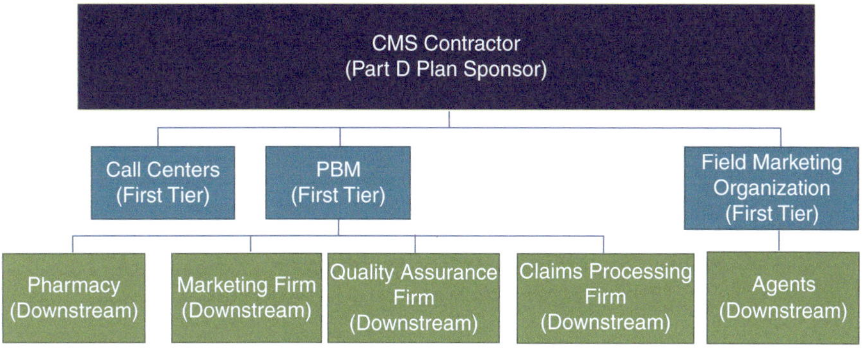

Fig. 8.1 Stakeholder relationships of Medicare Part D benefit

affiliate. However, sponsors may use FDRs for compliance activities, such as monitoring, auditing, and training.

CMS also performs several reviews and audits related to a PACE organization's Part D bid development:

1. Bid desk review: shortly after each year's bid submission deadline and before CMS approves each bid, they conduct a desk review of all Part D bids to ensure they comply with the CMS bid instructions. CMS may require a Part D sponsor to submit a revised bid in response to a desk review finding.
2. Bid audit: after CMS approves the Part D bids, they randomly select certain Part D sponsors for a more in-depth actuarial audit of the bid development. Historically, CMS has audited the bids of one or two PACE organizations each year. Part D sponsors must address any bid audit findings in the bid development for the following year.
3. Financial audit: in addition to the actuarial audits of the bid development, CMS audits the accuracy of the experience data (PDE, DIR, and non-benefit expenses) used to develop a Part D sponsor's bids. **Certified public accountants conduct these audits on approximately one-third of all Part D sponsors each year. Part D sponsors are required to submit a Corrective Action Plan for each financial audit finding.**

Pharmacists in PACE

Pharmacists play an important role in PACE. While they are not part of the CMS-defined PACE interdisciplinary team (IDT), they are often directly involved in the care of participants. Furthermore, they play important clinical, financial, and administrative roles.

The concept of having a pharmacist on staff at a PACE organization (PO) is relatively new. Prior to the inception of Medicare Part D in 2006, pharmacists were fewer and farther between. In these earlier years, pharmacists performed clinical-type roles for PO executives who felt the need to have a medication expert. These pharmacists had a focus of assisting prescribers at ensuring participants were receiving the most safe, effective, and cost-optimized medications. As the pharmaceutical field evolves and a larger portion of dollars is spent on specialized medication regimens, the role of the pharmacist has adapted and increased in presence.

PACE participants **utilize an average of 10–12 medications each day** (eight prescriptions per member per month for *Part D medications).***Many POs find that the best way to ensure proper and optimized medication regimens is for the pharmacist to perform manual reviews on each PO member**. Typically, these reviews are conducted on either an annual or a semi-annual basis. The outcome of these reviews usually results in a consultation with the in-house PACE prescriber. Reviews and/or consultations reduce unnecessary, potentially harmful, or high-cost medications (when a lower-cost alternative is available).

Besides medication reviews, **the PO pharmacists often contribute or actively participate in IDTs to help put the complex medication regimens into perspective**. Incorporating such questions as, "Are these medications still needed?", "Is the participant taking his or her medications as prescribed?" "Is he or she experiencing any side effects because of medication use or drug interactions?" "What are the contributing factors as to why s/he fails to come to the day center to pick up their medication?" "What are the participant's medication goals?", and "Are there opportunities for deprescribing?" results in more comprehensive care as well as risk reduction inherent to medication use.

There are many triggers for nonadherence of medications. Pharmacists are there to assist in triaging these concerns and provide innovative solutions that work for both the PACE team and participant.

Pharmacists also have a role in disease-state management, reducing overall costs for emergency department (ED) visits and hospitalizations. Specific disease states may include diabetes, heart failure, and asthma/chronic obstructive pulmonary disease (COPD), as well as antibiotic stewardship. **The extent to which a pharmacist can also prescribe directly for disease state management to assist in the goals of care is dependent on state regulations.**

Another reason a PO would consider hiring, contracting, or otherwise collaborating with a pharmacist is to be a liaison between the organization and the dispensing pharmacy. PACE participants are subject to the prescribing of high-cost medications and polypharmacy. A pharmacist plays a pivotal role in determining what medications are both safe and cost-effective while assisting PACE in the optimization of therapy. Having a greater understanding of the dispensing pharmacy operations while incorporating PACE knowledge into decision-making allows for the implementation of strategic pharmacy operations through project management.

With the enactment of Medicare Part D in 2006, a pharmacist's role became more relevant to the PO. Pharmacists were identified as being valuable to internal PO finance departments as well as actuaries in developing the annual plan bid (see details in the next section of this chapter). Tasks in which a pharmacist can spearhead Medicare Part D management for a PO include the organization of pharmacy claims, coordination with pharmacy benefit management (PBM) or third-party administrators, and reconciliation of the prescription drug event (PDE) with the Centers for Medicare and Medicaid Services (CMS).

Regulations and Plan Monitoring

Pharmacists assist POs with CMS plan audits, Part D 1/3 financial audits, and operational oversight as it relates to Medicare Part D regulations. ("Part D 1/3 audits" refers to the number of plan sponsors (1/3) that are audited by CMS each year.) Clinical comprehension is useful for chart reviews for a variety of requirements related to CMS audits. Data analytic skills can be further leveraged for ongoing monitoring in medication-related areas of risk, such as fraud, waste, and abuse reviews. Often, POs depend on pharmacist skills and expertise to develop PO medication-related policies and procedures relating to Part D regulations. By virtue of licensure, a PO pharmacist understands pharmacy regulation and the associated impact on the PO itself as well as those served by the PO.

Medicare Part D 1/3 financial audits include at least one-third of Part D organizations' financial records – including bids, data relating to Medicare utilization, and allowable costs under sect. 1858(c). Audit sections vary each year. They typically include drug utilization management, quality assurance, pharmacy access, coordination of benefits, true out-of-pocket (TrOOP) costs, claim processing, and payment. Depending on the PO program setup, any applicable formulary and pharmacy and therapeutics (P&T) committee information may also be audited. POs may employ or contract with pharmacists assisting in these functions and enhance their responsiveness to 1/3 financial audit requests. Ongoing pharmacist oversight of these areas and coordination with any applicable pharmacy benefit managers (PBMs) should assist organizations in preventing negative audit findings as well as in avoiding unnecessary monetary penalties. For instance, a regular review of prescription drug event (PDE) data claims for Part B vs Part D billing allows for the early detection of issues and prevents large monetary takebacks from CMS postaudit findings. Further cost savings associated with audit risk are outlined in the following section.

Cost Savings/Cost Avoidance and Therapeutic Interchange

For outpatient drug costs associated with PACE plans, there are two main areas of concern: Part B drug costs and Part D drug costs.

Medicare Part B drug costs will help with the PACE plan's financials as this comes from the capitated dollars. Reviewing where specialty drugs come from (e.g., system pharmacy vs. contracted pharmacy vs specialty pharmacy) and if a biosimilar is available can bring substantial savings to the plan. Having the pharmacist as part of the treatment plan before therapy starts will help obtain buy-ins from the participant and treating prescriber. Having a pharmacist review both medical and prescription claims for Medicare Part B drugs could bring a large return on investment.

Medicare reimburses direct Part D drug costs on a 1:1 basis if the PO remains within the projected bid amount. Pharmacists are uniquely capable of identifying cost savings associated with Medicare Part D. Looking at capsules vs tablets (e.g., venlafaxine ER), biologic agents (specialty drugs, insulin glargine), and half-tablet capabilities (e.g., sodium-glucose cotransporter-2 inhibitors) are great places to start. **Drug cost savings begin to impact the PO's finances when the PO is off by 5% or more of their bid projections. The pharmacist is in a position to identify opportunities early in the fiscal year and appropriately initiate interventions leading to successful program-wide savings**.

The one exception where medications usually coded as Medicare Part D will have cost savings that may impact the PO's overall budget is if the participant has Medicaid only. In a Medicaid-only participant, claims are part of the capitated budget. In other words, Medicaid claims are not submitted to Medicare through prescription drug event data (PDE). A pharmacist can help prioritize cost-saving opportunities, all while ensuring that the participants, as well as the PO, are not slighted.

Cost-saving opportunities may also reduce the risk to the PO during audits. For example, a pharmacist, as a PO initiative, may convert prescription lidocaine or diclofenac patchees to over-the-counter alternatives, resulting in reduction of any potentially unnecessary or questionable Medicare reimbursed claims while not negatively impacting the intended care. In turn, the OTC formulation is generally less costly compared to the prescription preparation.

Participant Adherence Assessment

Assessing the ability to self-manage and aiding in medication management are the fundamental roles of a PO pharmacist. Generally, PO pharmacies prepare medications in specialized packaging that promotes simplicity, resulting in better adherence to the complex regimen. Packaging can involve weekly to monthly preparations, with single- or multidose solutions. Pharmacists can assist in the progression from prescription vials to specialized packaging and medication dispensing systems. **Education provided by a PO pharmacist to a participant prevents confusion as well as misunderstandings about dosing and the use of medication assistance devices**. As an informal part of the IDT, PO pharmacists may also work with nursing and occupational therapy professionals in determining the best type of medication dispensing system to employ, given the individual participant.

Besides participant ability, there are a variety of access issues that affect participant adherence. Starting with pharmacy selection, PACE programs have options when it comes to pharmacy operational structures. These include mail-order programs, retail chains, hospital-based or health system pharmacies, and independent pharmacy delivery programs. Often, the choice of pharmacy operations may affect a participant's ability to self-manage medications based on their understanding of accessing medications through the system itself. Pharmacists can assist in educating participants to navigate the nuances of PACE pharmacy services.

The Evolving Role of the PO Pharmacist

The role of the PO pharmacist continues to evolve. As more specialty medications become approved, the unique characteristics as well as associated costs of medication increase the need for a medication expert. In addition, medication safety technology plays an increasingly important role within the PO, requiring the guidance of a well-trained pharmacist.

Summary

Medication use among PACE participants is a challenging aspect of caring for this vulnerable population of older adults. A well-trained pharmacist with a geriatrics focus is a vital member of the IDT, who can provide key clinical advice as well as guidance on finances and regulations. Expertise in Part D medication coverage in collaboration with CMS is an integral aspect of PACE operations and requires managerial knowledge and the ability to navigate different coverage aspects of medication within PACE (Part B vs Part D, Medicare or Medicaid only, among other nuances). There are many payment and regulatory aspects of the pharmacy benefit that require specialized knowledge and attention to detail to achieve successful outcomes.

Chapter 9
Core Components of the Typical PACE Center

Kristie Hartig, David Wensel, and Gwen Graddy-Dansby

The primary objective of Programs of All-Inclusive Care for the Elderly (PACE) is to enable older adults to remain living in the community and to avoid nursing home and hospital admission. All PACE programs adhere to a common set of federal regulations (CFR) which mandate a set of core services that align with the goal of managing health issues and maintaining function. There is a physical space, or "PACE Center," which is the focal point of these services. With some minor variation between sites, all operate an Adult Day Health Center (ADHC), a medical care practice, and a rehabilitation unit on this campus (See Fig. 9.1). In the chapter, we describe these three areas to illustrate the important functions and structure of each.

The PACE Adult Day Health Center

Overview of Adult Day Care

In the general population (non-PACE), adult day care is a benefit available for older adults and can be a source of support for family caregivers. Generally, **there are three types of adult day programs: social adult day care, adult day health care,**

K. Hartig (✉)
Community Nursing, Midland Care Connection, Inc, Topeka, KS, USA
e-mail: khartig@midlandcc.org

D. Wensel
TRU Community Care, Lafayette, CO, USA
e-mail: davidwensel@trucare.org

G. Graddy-Dansby
PACE Southeast Michigan, Dearborn, MI, USA
e-mail: Dr.Graddy@pacesemi.org

M. K. McNabney (ed.), *Community-Based Integrated Care for Older Adults*,
https://doi.org/10.1007/978-3-031-05137-1_9

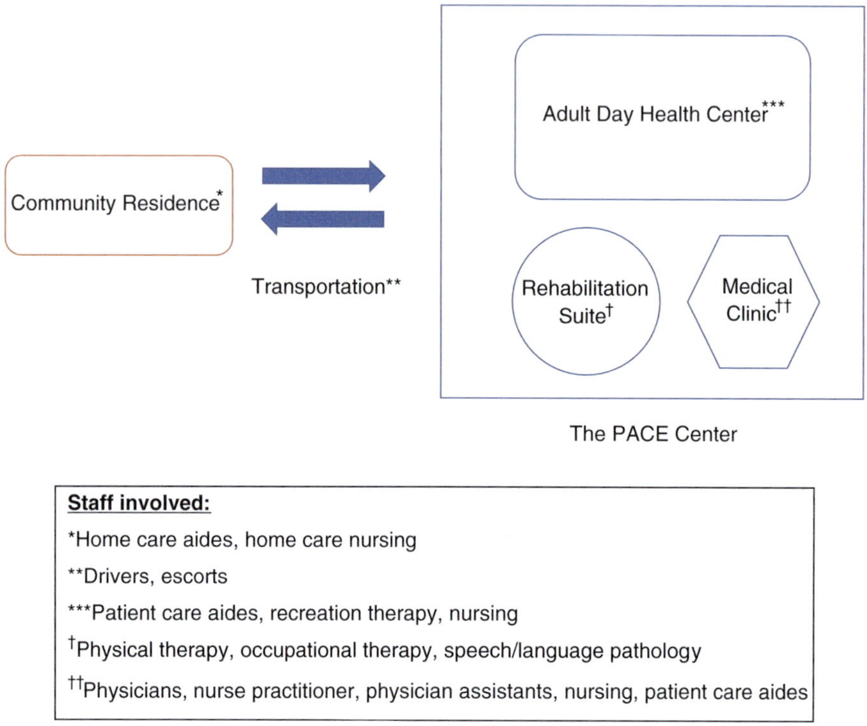

Fig. 9.1 The PACE Center

and specialized adult day care. Long-term care Medicaid in most states will provide funding assistance for individuals wishing to attend an adult care center under certain circumstances. In the past, long-term care Medicaid was provided only for those residing in a nursing home, but for older adults who qualify to live in a nursing home yet choose to stay in their own home, long-term care Medicaid waivers now allow for financial assistance with community services, including adult day care. There are multiple versions of the Medicaid waiver, and each state operates their Medicaid program a little differently, but those states that do not cover adult day care assistance through a Medicaid waiver typically have some other form of assistance or public funding for adult day care services. As of September 2019, all 50 states and Washington, DC offer assistance for adult day care in one form or another through their Medicaid programs [1]. The challenge for older adults who are not in a PACE program is that the availability of waivers is usually limited by enrollment caps or income limits for eligibility.

Adult day programs are considered a cost-effective way to manage the needs of many older adults with chronic diseases, allowing families to provide care to their loved ones at home instead of placing them in an institution. As previously mentioned, there are generally three types of adult day care, all of which provide daytime supervision of individuals in a group environment. General offerings of adult day service centers will include some form of meals and snacks, help with personal care, activities that encourage social interactions among individuals, and transportation to and from the center. Medicaid in each state may cover one type of adult day program but not the other, and although Medicaid in every state may pay for an adult care program, it is not always the best source of funding because the reimbursement rates are not high, and some adult day centers will not accept those individuals enrolled in Medicaid.

The first center type is the social adult day care (ADC). Services provided include non-medical supervision of recreational or social activities and healthy meal options. The next center type is the adult day health care (ADHC), sometimes referred to as adult day medical care, and this care program is mandated to provide a higher level of care and will have qualified nurses on staff that can assist with medical equipment, medication administration, personal hygiene, eating, dressing, transferring and mobility, and maintaining continence (or managing incontinence). Nutritious meals are provided along with social activities, and additional services may include speech therapy, physical therapy, or occupational therapy. The last program type is specialized adult day care, which has typically been available for Alzheimer's patients and those with varying forms of dementia. Specialized adult day care offers adult day health care services with the additional focus of preventing wandering, injuries, and challenges with behavior. Some centers will have all three program types available under one roof, but many individuals covered for these services through Medicaid have limits depending on the individual need, but no enrollee will exceed the maximum of 8 h per day and 5 days per week.

Each state determines the regulations for their adult day program models and depending on the state the center may require certification, licensure, or both. Federal guidance has been provided in the past through reports submitted by the Assistant Secretary for Planning and Evaluation (ASPE), the principal advisor to the Secretary of the U.S. Department of Health and Human Services. Each state has a definition of their adult day care models, and usually have their own criteria for individuals receiving services, restrictions on the number of hours an individual may receive services, and limitations on the number of participants that can be served at one time. Additionally, each state will make the determination of staffing licensure and training requirements as well as the number of staff required per number of participants.

The PACE Adult Day Program

PACE programs are federally regulated and there are specific mandates for PACE organizations (PO). A core service provided under the PACE model of care is adult day health care. **Every PO has a day health center (ADHC) that provides nursing, personal care, occupational therapy, physical therapy, recreational therapies, meals, nutritional counseling, and social work services**. Each state agency that administers the PACE program is in regular consult with the State Agency on

Aging. The size of the ADHC varies among locations but the focus is the same: delaying nursing home placement by keeping frail, elderly, qualifying individuals safely in their home. The use of the ADHC program offers increased supervision and assistance with chronic health care needs during the day.

The ADHC provides enhanced supervision capabilities for participants, all who require the level of care provided in a nursing facility. Caregivers are provided respite while the participant attends the ADHC, and they can also remain in the workforce while their loved one is provided care in the ADHC. Each PACE center is unique and readily adapts to the community it serves. Essential services are provided to participants with complex biopsychosocial and chronic health issues, enabling them to continue living alone in the community. Participants can attend the center 5 days per week but usually average 3 days a week, and transportation to and from the center is an included benefit with the PACE program. **Many participants are at the PACE center on a regular basis which contributes to the high volume of encounters a participant will have with a member of the interdisciplinary team**.

The **ADHC is located in the PACE center**, which also houses the medical clinic, staffed with a primary care medical provider. Participation in the day center allows for easy arrangement of in-clinic exams and follow up evaluations, thus, participants with acute problems such as COPD exacerbations, pneumonia or cellulitis can be rechecked daily, even receive intravenous (IV) therapies and blood draws, helping to avoid inpatient stays. Another benefit at the center is that medications are stored, administered, and distributed at the center. Medications are typically stored and provided to the participant per written prescription/ physician order. A licensed nurse or certified medication aide (CMA) may administer medication as ordered by the client's physician, but CMAs may be required to consult with a nurse prior to administering any PRN medications or insulin dosages based on blood glucose readings in some states.

The Adult Day Health Program provides a caring, secure environment for older adults. Through programming, medical services and peer socialization, the program strives to maintain the independence, dignity, and self-esteem of participants in the program. **ADHC staff may include a center manager, nurse, certified nurse aides and medication aides as well as recreation therapists. Chaplain and social worker are available as needed**. Participants must express need and desire for services, and all participants attending will have a Health Service Plan developed to reflect care needs. In the event the Functional Capacity Screen indicates that the client will need Health Care Services, a licensed nurse must assess the client and develop the health services plan.

Participants who participate in the ADHC are provided with a written guide of service needs, known as a Negotiated Service Agreement. The team is responsible for providing service(s) outlined and agreed to in the Negotiated Service Agreement, as determined via completion of the Functional Capacity Screen and development of the Health Service plan. Multiple factors are taken into consideration to optimize participant experience in the day center. Needs that are addressed include sensory, communication, physical abilities, cognitive status, psychological well-being, and program routines such as personal preferences, life enrichment program needs, task therapy, and habits or routines.

Summary

For older adults who can benefit from ADHC centers, having the day filled with social activities and a variety of interesting things to concentrate on will leave them feeling better. Research by the National Adult Day Services Association indicates that isolation can be as harmful to the human body as smoking tobacco. Using ADHC centers is the best way to prevent that additional harm from a loved one who is already in cognitive decline.

There are several benefits of a PACE ADHC program over a non-PACE program. Primarily, the PACE ADHC is an all-inclusive social and health services program. PACE provides comprehensive medical and supportive services across the entire continuum of care. By using these services, many older adults with chronic care needs who are enrolled in PACE are able to remain in their homes and maintain independence as long as possible.

The PACE Medical Clinic

Overview on General Medical Practices

In the general population (non-PACE), fee-for-service primary care practices for older adults are typically staffed by a physician provider (MD or DO), nursing support and office assistants. The physician might be board-certified in geriatric medicine, but that is uncommon. Frequently, such practices also utilize advance practice providers (nurse practitioners, physician assistants) and there is a high volume of patient visits per day (15 to 30-min visits are typical). There is broad mix of complexity among the patients seen; some very straight-forward ("well elderly") and some more complex. It is uncommon to have communication between outpatient providers and inpatient providers when patients are hospitalized. Non-PACE primary care practices have limited contact with patients between scheduled visits.

The PACE Medical Clinic

The Program of All-Inclusive Care for the Elderly (PACE) is responsible for all medical care provided to members of the program and the on-site medical clinic is a core component. It is the hub of medical care provision and coordination and also provides an opportunity for caregivers to interact with the PACE clinical teams, which consist of physicians, nurse practitioners, physician assistants, nurses, and medical assistants. This clinical team is responsible for providing all necessary medical care that is provided to PACE participants within the medical clinic and coordinating the management of all chronic medical conditions. PACE is the only model of care in the US that is at full risk for all needs of participants. When someone enrolls in a PACE, there is a consolidation of all Medicare benefits, and the PACE medical clinic becomes a major part of providing all needed medical services to participants. PACE medical providers also conduct house calls or home visits when needed, often with home care nurses or other members of the IDT (see Chap. 16). This is all coordinated by the PACE medical clinic. When PACE participants are seen in the medical clinic or on home visits, the medical providers do not bill Medicare for the individual visits as they operated with the capitated PACE reimbursement model. This allows providers to focus on management of their chronic medical conditions.

PACE medical clinics are very different than the usual Medicare fee-for-service (FFS) medical clinic. PACE clinics serve a very frail population who typically have multiple, chronic medical conditions. **PACE medical clinics attempt to provide all the necessary clinical services that a PACE participant might need to maintain health and medical stability in the community**. This typically includes all needed medical care, wound care, podiatry care, dental care, acute medical needs, chronic medical condition management, and other services as defined by the needs of the PACE population. Most traditional Medicare FFS medical clinics simply provide needed medical care and chronic disease management. In addition to these service, PACE medical clinics strive to minimize the need for participants to see providers (consultants) outside the PACE clinical teams and to also coordinate their care better. This helps to keep the PACE participant living independent and safe in the community. It also works to decrease the total number of medical providers caring for each PACE participant which helps to cut down on duplication of services and care. The PACE medical team and the care they provide through the PACE medical clinic is likely responsible for better medical outcomes and the ability of participants to live independently for a longer time in the community.

PACE medical clinics often have more access to participants and are therefore able to evaluate their medical needs quicker than a usual Medicare FFS medical clinic. Many participants attend the PACE Day Health Center frequently so that the PACE team can assist in their care. (See section on Day Health Center). This provides the opportunity for the PACE medical team to monitor the health of participants in a much closer way and treat urgent problems before they get worse. By having the medical clinic near the Day Health Center, PACE is better able to serve the participant and their medical needs often reducing the need for acute hospital visits and emergency department visits which can be very difficult for a PACE participant. This allows the PACE medical team to be very involved in the development of the care plan that is used to provide all the needed services to help PACE participants remain living independent in the community safely.

PACE medical clinics and the PACE medical providers do not bill Medicare for the individual clinical visits. A normal Medicare medical clinic will typically see at least one patient every 15 min and bill Medicare for each visit. The PACE medical team can spend more time with a participant since the visits are not billed on a per visit basis. Often the PACE medical team will see the participant along with the caregivers to address any questions or concerns. This allows the caregiver to also be involved in the medical care and the development of the care plan for the PACE participant. The PACE medical provider is often caring for a much smaller panel of patients than the usual Medicare provider. This allows the medical clinic and providers to address issues sooner before they become acute medical issues that require hospitalization. This often means a higher number of clinical encounters with any individual PACE participant if the need arises. It is much easier for a PACE participant to be seen in the PACE medical clinic for urgent needs than a usual Medicare participant can be seen in the typical Medicare medical clinic.

Most PACE participants have multiple chronic conditions that require regular management. They are often functionally impaired and require assistance with their activities of daily living (ADL). When the PACE medical team interacts with other interdisciplinary team (IDT) members, it allows them to become aware of small changes that other team members may have noticed. The PACE IDT consists of medical providers, nurses and nurses' aides, medical assistants, drivers, social workers, dieticians, physical therapist, occupational therapist, home health aides, adult day center staff, life enrichment, dieticians, and volunteers. This interaction allows the PACE medical team to address issues earlier in the PACE medical clinic than the usual Medicare Medical clinic that does not have access to an interdisciplinary team. Since the PACE IDT includes transportation, the PACE medical clinic can have a participant brought into clinic at any time. This flexible scheduling system with the assistance of an IDT can prevent small issues from becoming major medical problems leading to further functional decline in the participants. The PACE medical providers have more access to the participants, and this allows them to manage their chronic medical problems much closer than the usual medical clinic.

Most PACE medical clinics do not operate in a typical 9:00 to 5:00 model like a Medicare FFS medical clinic. The average PACE participant may not arrive at the PACE day health center until around 10:00. They will remain at the day center usually until around 15:00 so there may be a smaller window of time to see participants in the PACE medical clinic. For this reason, the daily clinic schedule may change based on the needs of individual PACE participants, and urgent medical problems that may have occurred in the last 24 h. **The PACE medical providers schedule is more flexible and follows a more open scheduling model to accommodate the urgent changes that may be needed**. This is often not possible in a Medicare medical clinic due to the number of patients being followed.

Another great advantage the PACE medical clinic has over the usual Medicare FFS medical clinic is the collaboration between the PACE medical team and the physical therapy and occupational therapy team members. The PACE clinical staff work closely with the therapy staff to evaluate and treat many of the same medical problems. Often the rehabilitation department (PT and OT) is located very close to the medical clinic so that team members can work together when needed. In the normal Medicare FFS medical model, the clinical staff very often do not communicate with the therapy staff and the patients do not receive the benefit of the teams working together to solve medical and functional issues before they get worse. **Since many of the PACE participants attend the Day Health Center multiple times a week, it is much easier to reschedule them to be seen later in the week**

rather than some time later in the month. This allows PACE participants to be seen more often when needed for complicated medical issues such as wound care, infections, Intravenous therapies, and acute medical issues that may help avoid hospitalizations and emergency department visits.

PACE medical clinics vary in size and capabilities based on the PACE census and building location. Some PACE clinics serve only a few participants, and some serve as many as several thousand participants (in multiple locations). Some PACE clinics serve very urban populations in large cities, while other serve very rural populations and are in smaller communities. For PACE centers that serve a large population, the Day Health Center may operate different shifts during a 24-h time period. In those cases, some of the PACE medical clinics work in different shifts to allow for more PACE participants to be seen when they come into the adult day center. The PACE medical provider is often caring for a much smaller panel of patients than the usual Medicare FFS provider. This allows the PACE medical provider to know the PACE participant in a more complete way. The PACE medical provider is usually caring for around 100 PACE participants where the usual Medicare FFS provider will have a panel size of 500 to 1000 patients.

PACE medical clinics are set up physically very similar to a traditional medical clinic with usual clinic rooms that have an exam table, sink, and desk. Many PACE clinics also have rooms dedicated to procedures with specialized chairs to accommodate functionally impaired patients. They will also have large scales to allow for participants to be weighed in a wheelchair. Some PACE medical clinics also have dental style chairs in rooms to allow for dentist to come into the clinic and provide oral care to participants. PACE medical clinics may have rooms with hospital beds and monitoring capabilities to provide more urgent care to patients who need additional care or who cannot tolerate a standard medical exam table. Another common difference between a PACE medical clinic and the standard medical clinic is the size of exam rooms; the PACE medical exam rooms are often larger to accommodate wheelchairs or other mobility assistance devices.

PACE medical clinics are able to adapt in support of the participant and the IDT. The PACE clinic may operate at any time during the day to allow for later hours. Many of the PACE participants will rely on the PACE transportation team to bring them into the Day Health Center and clinic. Participants may also need someone to come to the home and help them get ready for a visit and the timing of these visits may vary widely; the PACE medical clinic must allow for these changes to happen. Urgent medical issues can also arise, and this can slow down the clinic flow of participants. PACE participants will often be seen for urgent needs in the PACE medical clinic before going to the hospital or emergency department. Since most PACE participants attend the Day Health Center, regularly, it is very easy to postpone appointments or change them as needed.

Staffing PACE medical clinics varies between PACE programs based on the needs of that community. Most PACE clinics will have a medical assistant to help with getting PACE participants into the exam rooms and getting them ready for the provider visit. Some PACE clinics will also be staffed with Certified Medication Aides to help with medication administration at the Day Health Center and to help with other care as needed. Many PACE medical clinics will also have a Registered Nurse or a Licensed Practical Nurse available to provide advanced nursing services such as wound care, intravenous therapy, phlebotomy, medication administration, and assistance with office procedures. **This variety of staffing models allows PACE medical clinics to adapt and assist with the needs of the participants**. PACE medical clinics vary in size and scope with the ability to grow as the PACE program expands.

PACE medical clinics are designed to provide medical care to very frail, functionally impaired older adults who have complex medical issues. They are built for the care of this population which is very different than the usual Medicare FFS medical clinic space. The smaller panel sizes and ability to have longer medical visits, allows the medical provider to know the medical and psychosocial issues in greater depth. It is a better way to care for nursing home-eligible people who are still capable of living safely in the community with help. The PACE medical clinic operates to support this goal and care for participants up to the time of their death.

Summary

The PACE medical clinic is appropriately located in close proximately to the "social hub" of the participants attending the Day Health Center. This setting is quite conducive to arranging scheduled appointments for monitoring and treating chronic conditions as well as allowing for the "quick response" to acute and subacute changes that are noticed by the IDT in the DHC or in the home setting. PACE teams learn how to distribute clinical staff within the Center to optimize the ability to monitor health status and intervene appropriately.

The PACE Rehabilitation Suite

As the population continues to age, healthcare will be more challenged with how to maintain older adults safely at home in the community. One of the major reasons for placement in nursing homes is limitations or dependency in activities of daily living (ADL), such as dressing, bathing, toileting and walking. Rehabilitation services ("rehab") are used to improve or maintain functional status.

In "non-PACE" scenarios, the ability to get rehab services is complicated by significant paperwork. If outpatient referrals for rehab are made, there are no guarantee that these will be approved. Primary care physicians might request rehab services based on clinical assessment and judgment, yet the patient will not get therapy because "did not meet the criteria." In other scenarios, rehab might be initiated but stop because the patient did not appear to be making progress. However, a definition of progress can be "to improve/maintain independence enough to be safe in the home, relieve pain, maintain safe mobility to reduce the risk of a fall."

Rehabilitation specialists (occupational and physical therapists, in particular) are vital and necessary components of any care model that serves older adults. Rehab services really can make the difference in preventing a premature, permanent admission into a nursing home or an avoidable hospital admission. Therapists are capable and have the ability to help keep someone safe and independent in their home.

History of Rehabilitative Services

The use of rehabilitation as a means of promoting health is not a new concept. In fact, the word "therapy" comes from the ancient Hebrew word *refua* which means healing [1]. In the fifth century the Greek physician Herodicus described an elaborate system of gymnastic exercises for prevention and treatment of diseases. Also, around that time the ancient Chinese employed Cong Fu, as a movement therapy to relieve pain, not to be mistaken with Kung Fu the martial arts form. In the eighteenth century, Niels Stensen explored the biomechanics of human motion and how it impacted health while Joseph Clement Tissot developed the use of medical and surgical gymnastics to promote the value of movement as an alternative to bedrest for patients recovering from surgery, neurologic conditions and strokes. Even before physical and occupational therapy were established as types of rehabilitative care, the health benefits of structured movements and exercise had been well established.

During the First World War those who performed physical therapeutic interventions were known as "reconstructive aides." They were trained to help rehabilitate injured soldiers. Early occupational therapy also known as "reconstructive aides" gained popularity during WWI. They were primarily used to treat people with mental or emotional disorders.

The benefits of physical and occupational therapy continued to gain momentum in the twentieth century and is recognized as an established discipline and important member of the multidisciplinary care team (IDT) [2].

Members of Rehabilitation Team and Their Roles

The primary members of the rehabilitation team consist of a physical therapist, occupational therapist, physical and occupational assistants and speech therapist (also known as speech pathologist). Although physical therapy (PT) and occupational therapy (OT) are two distinct disciplines they are complimentary and more often than not work together on meeting the needs of the patient (see Chap. 19).

PT's focus is to restore motion, create mobility, relieve pain, and increase function.

OT's emphasis is to improve performance of daily tasks to maintain independent living.

Speech Language Pathology (SLP) works to prevent, assess, diagnose and treat speech disorders. It also helps to develop language, improve social and cognitive communication, and swallowing disorders.

Rehabilitation Services in a Traditional Non-PACE Model of Care

There are several aspects that differentiate Rehabilitative services in a traditional model (non- PACE) from a PACE model. **Location can determine the success or failure of the outcome of rehab**. In a non-PACE model rehab services can be provided in one of many locations: an acute inpatient setting, inpatient rehab unit, nursing facility, outpatient center, or home. Often location may be dependent on insurance coverage, nursing home ratings, and availability of beds. For example, during the COVID pandemic bed availability became a major barrier in being able to place patients who needed skilled rehab into facilities. Nursing facilities refused accepting new and, in some cases, established patients after a hospitalization if the patient was COVID positive. This left hospitals with having to provide alternatives to rehab. PACE was able to provide other options including converting PACE sites to COVID recovery units where all services could be provided including rehab services. Staff would also be able to provide more care in the home.

Next, **the duration of rehab is determined by the patient need based on the initial assessment by the rehab team and often the medical team input**. Unfortunately, too often the time allowed is not enough to get patients back to or even close to baseline. If they respond slowly or appear to have reached a plateau, rehab may be prematurely discontinued. If they are unable to participate for at least 3 h-a-day sessions patients are not a candidate for skilled inpatient rehab. The amount of time typically allotted may not be enough thereby placing the patient at risk for continued functional decline and possible permanent nursing home placement. I will share a case with you that demonstrates the importance of duration and its impact.

Finally, insurance coverage has limitations whether CMS or third-party insurance carriers determine the location of therapy and duration of therapy. For example, Medicare A covers certain conditions and for a limited time. This coverage is limited up to 100 days per each benefit period. Medicare will cover a short-term stay in a Medicare-certified skilled nursing facility. The first 20 days are fully covered, the patients may have to pay a co-pay for continuation of rehab services during days 21–100. Beyond 100 days there are several options: pay out of pocket, wait until there is availability in the next benefit period, be discharged home or convert to a basic bed in the nursing home. This can be repeated after 60 days. Another limiting factor is in order to qualify for skilled rehab in a nursing facility the patient must be in the hospital for at least 3 days or 30 days after the hospitalization and require skilled services for the condition that was treated during the hospitalization. A patient would not typically be able to go directly from home to a skilled bed in a nursing facility even if the skilled level of rehab was needed.

In summary, receiving rehab services in a traditional non-PACE model can be limiting. This is a complicated set of factors which can have a negative impact on a patient's overall outcomes, ability to remain home and quality of care.

Rehabilitation Services at the PACE Center

It is important to understand the full impact that PACE rehab services have on the participants who enroll into PACE.

One of the criteria to be eligible for PACE is to meet a nursing home level of care, and one of the most common reasons for older adults in the community to need nursing home level of care is dependence in Activities of Daily Living (ADL). Approximately one-third of people admitted into long term care facilities are dependent in 3 or more ADLs. Furthermore, the people who are permanent residents of nursing home are at risk of increased dependence which further reduces the likelihood of returning to their home in the community.

The interdisciplinary team IDT is the foundation of PACE effectiveness, which includes the rehab team (PT and OT). From the time of enrollment, the important role of rehab is stressed for all PACE participants.

Dependence in ADLs is a marker for frailty, hospitalizations and nursing home placement.

National statistics show 86% of all PACE participants require some assistance with ADLs [3].

Proactive and prompt interventions will help avoid at-risk outcomes of this population.

Irrespective of where rehab occurs, PACE (insurer) and the provider continue to be involved in the participant's care. The rehab team communicates with the inpatient rehab team and nursing facility team. If it is decided that PACE can provide rehab in lieu of a nursing home facility or even inpatient rehab—PACE coordinates, develops and carries out the plan of care. This allows for continuity since PACE is already familiar with the participant and knows the pre-hospital or pre-event status. It brings value to an inpatient rehab team to be able to get baseline information on a participant from a similar discipline who speaks the same language. In addition, the PACE rehab team not only knows the participant but they also have information on their home environment and other facts are helpful in deciding about where rehab should be provided. E**ach PACE site has a dedicated rehab area that is staffed with PT, OT and assistants. All core equipment needed to perform a full scope of services is on-site**.

Having no limits on how many days, weeks or months rehab is provided can be extremely beneficial to a participant's outcome. Centers for Medicare & Medicaid Services (CMS) gives PACE the leverage for the IDT to make the right decisions that impact participant care. The provider does not have to worry about putting in a referral and waiting for approval because the rehab team has already done the assessment and brings their findings and recommendations back to the provider. However, if the provider wants a participant seen for whatever reason it is simply a call, email, walk into the rehab area, or a face-to-face conversation. No red tape, no delays. Next, **there is no end date for rehab as with traditional models**. The duration is determined by the need, benefit to participant, availability and willingness of both staff and participant to participate. The IDT has the leverage to plan, make decisions and carry them out based on what is RIGHT for the participant. This takes us into the next factor that impacts rehab services.

Insurance coverage in PACE as it relates to rehab services really has no limitations. The discussion may start in the IDT. Rehab evaluates, completes an assessment and a decision is made. As it relates to location, if a participant is in a nursing home and they have used up their Medicare A days, the rehab teams recommends that the participant would benefit from more skilled rehab. There are three options: approve additional days in the nursing facility, bring them into the center for additional skilled rehab, or send them home and provide the additional rehab either in the home or in the center. There are no limitations or restrictions on providing care if the rehab team deems it necessary. Their focus for the participant is always on safety, returning to the community and if return to the home is not an option and sometimes it is not, maximize independence. Another benefit of PACE is there is no minimum length of stay in hospital requirement to be eligible for admission into a skilled rehab. PACE has a waiver which allows them to not only bypass the 3-day hospital stay but to also admit directly from home for skilled rehab. PACE as the insurance company can approve up to 100 days and more if needed.

Who Gets Rehab Services in PACE?

This starts with an initial evaluation and often includes an in-home assessment. A recommendation from the rehab team comes from their assessments and information from other members of the IDT. Following the assessment, a care plan is developed which includes the assessment and the identified needs, a plan for providing the care as well as frequency of services and participant preferences. The IDT is also kept informed of how the participant is doing and any changes which is important for other members of the IDT. Another important difference is that the referral or recommendation for rehab involvement is not limited to the primary care physician or other providers. Any member of the IDT or staff that identifies or suspects a problem can report to the rehab team and the participant will be seen and evaluated. This is a great benefit because it is real time. It eliminates the need for referral and approval. The fact that the participant is known by the rehab team beyond their rehab needs is another benefit. In other words, the participant is not just a rehab client.

For example, a participant joins PACE and is assessed by the rehab team and a plan is developed. If a participant is not progressing or participating in rehab services, this information is brought back to the IDT. The participant's social worker may get involved to see if there are other things occurring in the participant's life that may be impacting their ability to participate. The rehab team can now incorporate this into how they relate to the participant. Another important difference between non-PACE and PACE rehab is they physically go into the participants' homes. This allows environmental assessment modifications all aimed at keeping the participant safe at home.

Education and training are given on durable medical equipment (DME) which is necessary to assure that it is being used safely. The coverage for DME in non-PACE is determined by the insurance, however, if the PACE rehab team deems it appropriate PACE will provide that piece of equipment. Every participant that enrolls in PACE is assessed by the rehab team every 6 months or when there is a change. An example of a change is when a participant has a fall. There is a post-fall evaluation in the center and depending on where the fall occurs an in-home visit may be required.

Finally, it is safe to say that the doors to the rehab department are literally open to all who enroll into PACE. Rehab services plays an important role in keeping PACE participants safe and independent in the community.

The case of Mr. Z is from PACE SEMI and highlights the multifaceted approach by PACE and its amazing rehab team.

Patient Story

Mr. Z enrolled in our PACE program late 2018. He is a 62-year-old who presented with significant history of orthopedic limitations and prior surgeries affecting his shoulders, spine, hips, and knees. Despite these complications, Mr. Z lived alone in a senior apartment, he utilized crutches to ambulate a short distance in his apartment and used a wheelchair for community distance.

This participant's fragile condition deteriorated rapidly requiring emergency spinal surgery involving thoracic through sacral regions on 3/28/2019. Subsequently, he was transferred from the hospital to subacute rehab. He required a 2–3 person assist with transfers, was unable to bear weight, and required maximum assistance with self-care activities while in bed. He was discharged from subacute rehab after only 2 weeks due to "lack of progress" and a recommendation of long-term care placement was rendered.

The PACE rehab team collaborated with the participant and other IDT members to transfer him to a nursing home in the Dearborn, MI catchment area which was closer to the PACE center that he had attended prior to the hospitalization and to maximize his ability to attend our center for rehab. Then PACE SEMI rehab team worked closely with the PACE transportation department to provide safety education, training and problem solving to ensure both participant and staff safety during the transportation route and loading/unloading onto the van.

After residing in a nursing home for 8 months in a basic bed and receiving 3 to 5 days a week and 1 to 3 h a day of therapy, with both PT and OT, this participant functionally progressed to the extent that he was able to be discharged to a wheelchair accessible apartment. To his credit, he remained highly motivated to improve.

Currently Mr. Z lives alone and is safe in the community with PACE services including, but not limited to, meals and home care services. Our PACE social worker played a major role in finding suitable housing for the participant. Without PACE and the unlimited rehab services, this participant most likely would have been in a nursing home for the rest of his life.

The rehab team are quick to admit that it took an entire team to make this happen, participant care assistants, social workers, nursing and transportation. Every member had a role, but the rehab team led the charge.

This story happened because of the PACE rehab team and its ability to collaborate with other disciplines to give this participant another chance at life.

This could not have happened without removing limits that can prevent needed rehab. As a result, quality of life is improved and a participant can return independently to the community.

Summary

The role of rehabilitation services in PACE takes on a more integrated role than what one would expect in the non-PACE world. Although PACE rehab services cover all of the traditional services provided by non-PACE rehab services, PACE rehab has a different focus allowing them to provide a greater range of care.

Rehab services are a part of the integration that is required to keep participants functional, independent and safe in their homes. They are the spokes that keeping the wheels of participants active and moving. One of the favorite areas for participants enrolled in PACE is rehab. They go to ride a stationary bike, get a heat pack, get on the parallel bars, and practice the correct way to use the walker or just socialize with other participants. It is therapeutic in many ways beyond the rehab services.

General Summary: The PACE Center

This chapter has highlighted one the primary strengths of the PACE model – "one-stop shop" of the PACE Center. Indeed, this focus of service truly captures the combined strengths of this community-based, integrated care model. The social atmosphere of the Adult Day Health Center creates a place of community and connection that provides many direct and indirect benefits to participants. The co-location of the rehabilitation services and medical services allows for highly efficient and proactive use of services that are so necessary to preserve function and health status in a select population of older adults who are otherwise vulnerable to decline in function, destabilization of medical problems and greater likelihood of hospitalization and nursing home care. The PACE Center is the "home" of the interdisciplinary team that pulls all of this expertise together to allow for better outcomes.

References

1. Caring.com. Paying for seniors: Understanding your financial options for long term care. Paying for Senior Care. 2020. https://www.payingforseniorcare.com/medicaid-waivers/adult-day-care. Accessed 11 Sept 2021.
2. Expand your circles prevent isolation and loneliness as you age [Pamphlet]. 2018. The Administration for Community Living. https://eldercare.acl.gov/public/resources/brochures/docs/Expanding-Circles.pdf
3. Careasone. The 3 types of adult day care. n.d. https://careasone.com/blog/the-3-types-of-adult-day-care/. Accessed 11 Sept 2021.

Suggested Reading

1. Burrows A, DeGolia P, Wensel D, editors. PACE medical directors handbook. 3rd ed. Alexandria, VA: National Pace Association; 2018.
2. Medicare and Medicaid Programs; Programs of All-Inclusive Care for the Elderly (PACE); Program Revisions, 71 F.R. 71244 (Dec. 8, 2006) (to be codified at 42 C.F.R. pt. 460, 462, 466, 473, and 476).
3. National Adult Day Services Association. About adult day services. n.d. https://www.nadsa.org/learn-more/about-adult-day-services/. Accessed 11 Sept 2021.
4. Oliver RE, Foster MA. Adult day care: an important long-term care alternative & potential cost saver. Mo Med. 2013;110(3):227–30.
5. Mayo Clinic Staff. Adult day service: What you need to know. 2020. https://www.mayoclinic.org/healthy-lifestyle/caregivers/in-depth/adult-day-service/art-20044261. Accessed 11 Sept 2021.
6. Morris S. 3 types of adult day care. n.d. https://www.agingcare.com/articles/types-of-adult-daycare-191250.htm. Accessed 11 Sept 2021.
7. Kansas Department for Aging and Disability Services. Community services FAQS. n.d. https://kdads.ks.gov/commissions/commission-on-aging/aging-and-disability-resource-centers/service-information/community-services. Accessed Sept 2021.
8. Segal J, Robinson L, White M. Adult day care services. 2020. https://www.helpguide.org/articles/senior-housing/adult-day-care-services.htm. Accessed 11 Sept 2021.
9. Schmitt EM, Sands LP, Weiss S, Dowling G, Covinsky K. Adult day health center participation and health-related quality of life. Gerontologist. 2010;50(4):531–40. https://doi.org/10.1093/geront/gnp172.
10. SNF Care Coverage (medicare.gov). https://www.medicare.gov/coverage/skilled-nursing-facility-snf-care. Accessed 2 Feb 2022.

Part IV
The PACE Team and Essential Roles

Chapter 10
The Interdisciplinary Team and Process in PACE

Becket Lauten and Lori Calkins

The use of this team-based approach to care delivery began in the United States over 100 years ago. In the early part of the twentieth century, Dr. Richard Cabot of Massachusetts General Hospital recognized that social factors had a significant impact on the health of his patients, and therefore were worthy of attention. He advocated for the inclusion of social workers, nurses and chaplains working with physicians to address nonmedical issues [1]. Dr. Martin Cherkasky at New York City's Montefiore Hospital advanced this model in 1948 when he created an outreach program which sent teams of physicians, nurses, and social workers to deliver home-based care to patients in the community [2].

The use of IDTs in care delivery gained momentum in the late 1960s, when the Office of Economic Opportunity provided funding for the development of community health centers throughout the US [2]. These health centers largely utilized a team approach in delivering care to patients. The Department of Veterans Affairs launched Home Based Primary Care in 1972 to deliver comprehensive care to Veterans with chronic medical and behavioral health conditions. Today, this program supports Veterans throughout the country. Care is coordinated and delivered by interdisciplinary teams with the goal of supporting Veterans to remain in the community, avoid institutionalization, and experience an improved quality of life [3].

The interdisciplinary approach is not unique to healthcare. Educational institutions have long utilized this model of instruction in medicine and science to broaden students' critical thinking skills [4]. In this model, students gain knowledge from

B. Lauten (✉)
Social Work, Providence ElderPlace, Portland, OR, USA
e-mail: becket.lauten@providence.org

L. Calkins
Nursing/Operations, Providence ElderPlace, Seaside, OR, USA
e-mail: lori.calkins@providence.org

M. K. McNabney (ed.), *Community-Based Integrated Care for Older Adults*,
https://doi.org/10.1007/978-3-031-05137-1_10

various disciplines allowing them to gain a breadth of understanding in areas that would likely not be possible from single-subject study [5]. Environmental projects have used interdisciplinary management to integrate the work of various disciplines in sustainability developments such as water resource projects [6]. Bringing together various disciplines to address a problem or need creates an opportunity for the integration of a variety of perspectives, thus resulting in a more well-rounded solution. The benefits of an interdisciplinary approach and how it provides more comprehensive, person-centered care for older adults enrolled in a PACE program will be explored further in this chapter.

IDT membership is determined by the needs of the program which it supports, as well as by regulatory directives. IDTs can vary in structure, from just a few members to a dozen professionals working together. A typical hospice IDT consists of a medical director, primary care provider, nurse case manager, social worker, chaplain, and a certified nursing assistant—all of which are roles mandated by the Medicare Hospice Benefit [7]. The focus of the hospice IDT is to alleviate suffering for those who are determined to be in the last 6 months of life and no longer seeking curative treatments. An IDT in a stroke rehabilitation setting may include a physician, nurse, and social worker, with the addition of occupational, physical and speech therapy professionals and a clinical psychologist [8]. These disciplines are selected for their expertise in helping patients regain functioning after a stroke. While federal regulations inform the composition of an IDT, the needs of its target population are also considered so that the team is prepared to provide care that is most relevant to the needs and goals of its population.

The IDT in the PACE Model of Care

Today's PACE model of care grew out of a community's desire to develop culturally appropriate services for older adults in San Francisco's Chinatown. Marie-Louise Ansak, a social worker, and Dr. William Gee, a dentist, were asked to consult on the development of a nursing facility for older adults in the community. Instead, inspired by a suggestion from a geriatrician from England, they developed a day center, On Lok, where seniors could go to receive medical and social services during the day and return home to their families in the evening [9]. This model, based on the British concept of the day hospital, allowed frail older adults to receive the support and services they needed to maintain independence and remain living in community-based settings [10]. **From the beginning, On Lok utilized an interdisciplinary approach to provide care that met the medical and social needs of its clients**. Nearly 50 years after On Lok opened its doors, 264 PACE sites throughout the nation continue to delivery comprehensive care to older adults through IDTs [11].

The IDT in a PACE program is responsible for developing a care plan for the participant, in the parlance of the PACE model. The guiding principles in every care plan are the goals, values and wishes of each participant. When these elements guide the development of the care plan, person-centered care is the result. The care plan developed by the IDT reflects that which is important to the participant, therefore each care plan is as unique as the individual it supports.

A care plan is developed through the work of individual IDT members completing their discipline-specific assessments for each participant. Assessments are completed when a participant enrolls in the PACE program and every 6 months, and these assessments are integrated into a care plan which documents the support that will be provided for the participant (see Chap. 21). The care plan aligns with the participant's goals and wishes and can be modified as needed as the participant's goals evolve—for example, if someone opts to no longer pursue curative interventions but wishes to focus on palliative care.

The disciplinary makeup of the IDT (see Fig. 10.1) is mandated by the Centers for Medicare & Medicaid Services (CMS), the division of the federal government which oversees Medicare and Medicaid programs and health plans that are funded by these entities (see Chap. 7). **PACE is funded by Medicare and Medicaid, and therefore IDTs must be comprised of the following disciplines**:

- Primary care provider (MD/DO, NP, PA).
- Nurse.
- Center manager.
- Occupational therapist.
- Physical therapist.

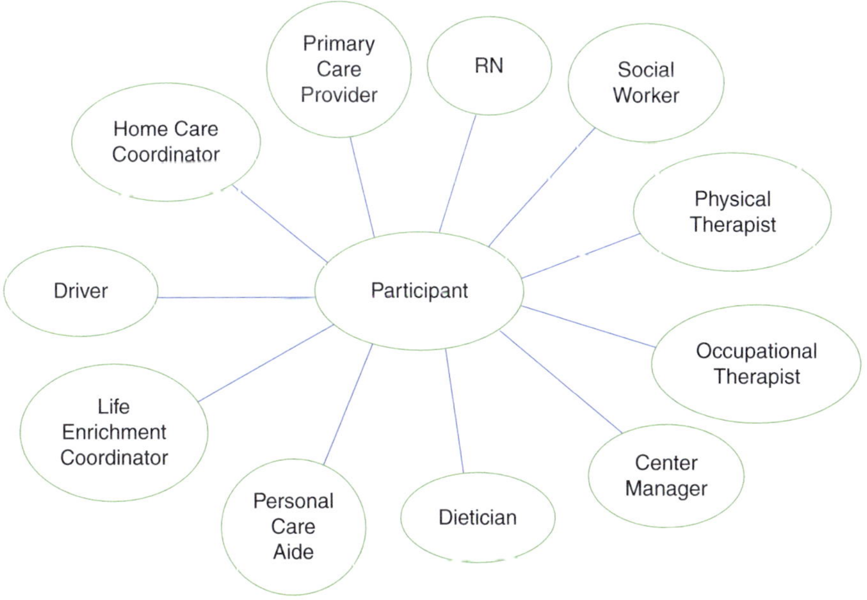

Fig. 10.1 IDT composition at Providence ElderPlace, Portland, OR. (Modified from a diagram in Nash, M. & Foidel, S. (2019). *Neurocognitive Behavioral Disorders: An Interdisciplinary Approach to Patient-Centered Care*. Springer 2018. Copyright Maureen C. Nash, MD. 2018 Fig. 2.2, pg. 52)

- Social worker.
- Van/bus driver.
- Personal care aide.
- Home care coordinator.
- Activity coordinator.
- Dietician.

While these are the disciplines that CMS requires at a minimum to participate in the IDT [12], PACE programs often operate with additional disciplines on their IDTs based on the needs of their participants.

These 11 disciplines contribute to the IDT meeting, but only eight are required to complete initial assessments of new participants enrolling in the PACE program [13]. The Primary Care Provider, Nurse, Social Worker, Physical Therapist, Occupational Therapist, Dietician, Life Enrichment Coordinator (activities coordinator), and Home Care Coordinator complete their discipline specific assessments while remaining attentive to the participant's goals and values—the focal point of the care planning process. A participant is actively engaged in the assessment process to the greatest extent possible, but the provider will also look to other resources in working to understand what is important to a participant. This is especially true for participants with a cognitive impairment who are unable to provide an accurate history. Providers will reach out to family members, formal and informal care givers, and other involved supports to gather collateral information to develop a more robust assessment.

A well-informed, person-centered care plan cannot be developed if the IDT members only seek to understand the medical issues that are important to a participant, as has traditionally been the focus of primary care. Team members will seek to learn about the participant's history including their family composition, education, career, hobbies, spiritual values, cultural identity, exposure to trauma, and other factors that contribute to knowing the person as a whole [14]. The typical PACE IDT is comprised of the disciplines listed in the following section. Their function within the IDT and how they contribute to the development of a meaningful, person-centered care plan are described below. A more thorough description of the disciplines and their roles will be presented in the following chapters.

PACE Interdisciplinary Team

Primary Care Provider

The primary care provider (PCP) role can be filled by an MD, a DO, or a nurse practitioner. The PCP gathers medical history, completes a full initial and ongoing physical assessment, and seeks to gain an understanding of the participant's values around health care. Knowing the participant's attitudes toward health care and their past experiences can help lay a foundation of trust between the provider and the participant. The PCP also participates in discussions around goals of care so that the IDT can understand if the participant wishes to pursue longevity, function, or palliative care.

Registered Nurse

The RN role functions as a Case Manager, coordinating care, ensuring appropriate supplies are in place, conducting routine assessments, providing care such as wound management, and managing chronic conditions such as COPD and diabetes. At the typical PACE site, Clinic RN Case Managers see participants at the Day Health Center, while Community Care RNs (CCRNs) see participants in their home settings. CCRNs conduct episodic visits and report findings and outcomes to the Clinic RNs, thereby assuring continuity of care and ensuring that the team has the most updated clinical picture of the participant.

Social Worker

The Social Worker is responsible for gathering biopsychosocial information that helps the IDT understand the social and emotional factors that are important to the participant. A participant's history, values and goals are elicited in a Social Worker's initial assessment, and this information helps to develop a care plan that addresses not only presenting medical issues, but non-medical factors which can impact the participant's sense of well-being. The Social Worker also participates in goals of care conversations and assists with advance care planning. The Social Worker is responsible for representing the participant's perspective and wishes, and advocates both within the program and with external partners to ensure the participant's needs are met.

Physical Therapist

The Physical Therapist (PT) assesses the participant's mobility needs and ensures that they have the needed equipment to achieve maximum functioning, as well as a treatment plan that supports their goals. The PT develops a plan of care based on the participant's needs and goals, whether it be to increase functional independence or decrease pain. PTs also work with care providers in home settings and community-based care facilities to problem-solve mobility issues related to needs such as transferring and bathing. PTs monitor participants through ongoing assessment to determine the need for changes to the care plan if a participant's functional status changes due to a medical event.

Occupational Therapist

The Occupational Therapist (OT) reviews the participant's living setting to determine needed equipment or environmental modifications to improve safety and functioning in activities of daily living (ADLs). This includes offering weighted utensils which can help a participant with motor skill deficits eat independently or providing vision aids for someone with impaired vision. The OT also assesses for needs related to safety such as a participant's risk to fall or elope from a care setting and ensures that the care plan addresses mitigation of these safety concerns.

Center Manager

The Center Manager is responsible for the overall operations of the PACE Day Health Center. In addition to ensuring regulatory compliance, managing the center budget, and staffing allocations, the Center Manager facilitates IDT meetings and advocates for stewardship in the allocation of resources such as during discussion around nursing facility stays. The Center Manager ensures that staff have the tools they need to be effective in their roles and keeps staff up to date on new policies and practice changes. The Center Manager is also responsible for responding to grievances filed by participants or their representatives.

Dietician

The Dietician ensures that the participant and their caregivers have support and education around dietary practices that will help meet nutritional goals. The Dietician assesses the participant's needs around dietary texture to determine if a modified diet is needed, as well as nutritional status so that dietary supplements can be supplied if indicated. A participant's ability to eat and swallow is also monitored by the Dietician who will make a referral to Speech Therapy for follow-up if concerns arise.

Personal Care Aide

The Personal Care Aide (PCA) probably has the most contact with participants of any discipline at the Day Health Center. When a participant arrives at the Day Health Center, the PCA assists with escorting them into the building, taking vital signs and helping them get settled in the day room. PCAs help participants during their day center visits with ADL needs such as feeding and toileting, and often assist with recreational activities. Because the time PCAs spend with participants and how well they get to know them, the PCAs are often the first to notice a change in a participant which requires follow up from another discipline. PCAs regularly communicate changing participant needs to RNs, Social Workers, PTs, and others based on their regular observations.

Life Enrichment Coordinator

The Life Enrichment Coordinator (LEC), also called Activities Director or Recreation Director, assesses the participant's social and recreational needs through the lens of past and current interests. In their initial assessment, the LEC elicits the participant's values, how they prefer to socialize, any hobbies they used to or currently enjoy, and collaborates with other disciplines to determine if any sensory limitations might require modification of activities. LECs communicate with family members and caregivers to gather information on past interests for participants who are not able to participate in the assessment due to cognitive impairment. Recreational plans are then developed to include meaningful activity that is within the participant's abilities.

Driver

The Driver ensures that the participants arrive safely to the Day Health Center, as well as to outside specialty medical appointments. Drivers are the first point of contact in a participant's day, so they often receive information from caregivers that is passed on to other disciplines for follow-up at the Day Health Center. It is not uncommon for a Driver's observations of a participant's apparent change in mood or functioning to lead to further assessment by a clinician on the IDT.

Home Care Coordinator

The Home Care Coordinator (HCC) assesses the need for care for participants who live in independent settings and receive caregiving assistance from in-home providers. The HCC's assessment reviews the needs of the participant and the availability of natural supports to determine the allocation of caregiving hours that will be provided for the participant. The HCC also monitors the living settings of participants in community-based care settings to determine if added supports are needed.

There are other disciplines not required by CMS regulations but considered necessary, based on participant needs are active in both the IDT process and care plan development. For example, at some PACE programs, the Chaplain is involved for participants needing support with spiritual matters, and a Psychiatric Mental Health Nurse Practitioner and Mental Health Case Manager participate if there are behavioral health needs.

Interdisciplinary Team Meetings

PACE programs convene regular interdisciplinary team (IDT) meetings to coordinate the care of participants. These typically include ***daily brief team meetings*** which address key issues that arise and must be addressed promptly. These meetings are often called "stand up" or "morning" meetings" and comprised of those disciplines on duty on a particular day. There are also ***regularly scheduled (often weekly) IDT meetings*** which provide team perspective on treatment decisions and goals of care, as well as utilization management. The more formal ***interdisciplinary care plan (ICP) meetings*** typically occur weekly and require the participation of all 11 disciplines. Together, as a team, all disciplines share participant information, make determinations about services that will be provided, and monitor participant progress. Decisions made in the formal ICP meeting determine the individual participant care plan. Meetings are led by a facilitator, often the PACE Center Manager, who keeps the meeting discussion on task and encourages participation from all present. A scribe records the meeting discussion and reviews attendance to ensure that all required disciplines are present.

Decision-making around the provision of services or supplies is the responsibility of the entire IDT [14]. A PT may recommend that a participant be provided with a specialized piece of equipment, or a participant may request dentures during a visit with their RN. Those recommendations are brought to the IDT meeting for all disciplines to discuss and approve or deny. The benefit of the full IDT taking part in decision-making around participant needs and requests is that team members bring their discipline-specific perspectives to the discussion. In the example of the request for dentures, the RN will know to check in with the participant to ensure that the new dentures are not causing pain, and the Dietician will know to review the diet texture for any needed changes once the participant has adjusted to eating with dentures. These different perspectives ensure that an issue is addressed holistically, rather than from the view of just one just one discipline.

Elements of an Effective IDT

It is imperative that the team members arrive to the meeting prepared. Meetings have full agendas and team members have busy schedules, and preparation will ensure an efficient meeting. If someone brings a participant request to the meeting, they need to be able to speak concisely about the request, have all the relevant facts and be knowledgeable about policy related to the request. A recommended practice is for IDT members to bring requests to the team in SBAR (Situation, Background, Assessment, Recommendation) format. This model of communication ensures that everyone in the meeting will have the information they need to make an informed decision.

Participation is essential in a highly performing team. IDT meetings can be an intimidating venue for someone who is not comfortable speaking up in a large group. When requests are being discussed and decisions are being made, it is not a true interdisciplinary process if all team members do not participate. A team member who is not inclined to speak up in a large setting may hold a piece of information that could significantly impact the IDTs' decision-making process. **Full participation is necessary to ensure that all perspectives are bringing their expertise to the needs of the participant**.

The quality of team facilitation determines the effectiveness of an IDT. Facilitators are responsible for leading the meeting, ensuring required disciplines are present, and making sure that all items needing to be discussed are covered. A good facilitator keeps the discussion moving along and on topic. They also encourage full participation and remind attendees of expectations such as avoiding side conversations. PACE programs provide facilitator training and support to team members who wish to take on the facilitation role.

Potential Problems with the IDT Process

Even the most highly performing IDT can encounter challenges that if left unchecked, can undermine the effectiveness of the team process and trust among its members. **Poor professional boundaries, a lack of mutual respect among team members, and being unwilling to consider others' viewpoints are problems that would be apparent to most observers**. Less obvious issues can arise, however, and are sometimes not initially noticed even by the team members themselves. At times, the team cannot come to a decision about the right course of action regarding a participant's need, and some team members may feel distress around one or both of the possible outcomes. An ethics consultation will offer the IDT an opportunity for a focused discernment of the team's concerns and may alleviate some of the distress. Similarly, a team may be unable to agree on a clinical course of action, and a clinical consult involving the Medical Director and other individuals outside of the IDT may bring some direction to the team.

Tension between disciplines can arise in most IDTs and can be seen as detrimental to the team process. This tension arises from team members bringing their discipline-specific perspectives to an issue. Each member's perspective will bring them to view the issue differently, and where one team member sees a problem, another may see opportunity. A situation that illustrates this dynamic is a participant's wish to leave a supervised community-based living setting, such as an assisted living or residential care facility, and move in with an adult child who will provide care. A Social Worker would likely be in favor of supporting this choice based on their professional imperative of supporting participant choice and autonomy, while other disciplines might have some reservations. An OT might have concerns about the safety and accessibility of the home, and an RN might worry about the participant's ability to correctly take medications while their child is at work. **The tension between autonomy and safety is not necessarily harmful to the team process but rather a challenge to the team members to think creatively about how to minimize risk in this setting while supporting participant choice**.

Summary

In the PACE model, the IDT is responsible for supporting participants not only from a medical and functional perspective but also in the context of social and emotional needs. The PCP, RN, Social Worker, PT, OT, and other disciplines gain a deep understanding of their participants' needs and goals through the assessment process. A care plan is developed out of these assessments, and this care plan reflects the goals and values of the participant. An effective, highly functioning IDT empowers team members to provide person-centered care which reflects these goals and values while also challenging them to work through complex situations in an environment of support and mutual respect.

References

1. Dodds TA. Richard Cabot: medical reformer during the Progressive Era (1890–1920). Ann Intern Med. 1993;119:417–22.
2. Baldwin DC Jr. Some historical notes on interdisciplinary and interprofessional education and practice in health care in the USA. J Interprof Care. 2007;21:23–37.
3. Gillespie SM, Manheim C, Gilman C, et al. Interdisciplinary team perspectives on mental health care in VA home-based primary care: a qualitative study. Am J Geriatr Psychiatry. 2019;27:128–37.
4. Baldwin DC Jr, Baldwin MA. Interdisciplinary education and health team training: a model for learning and service. J Interprof Care. 2007;21:52–69.
5. Rahal L, Vadeboncoeur JA, PhD. Interdisciplinarity. Hackensack, NJ: Salem Press Encyclopedia; 2019.
6. Lanier AL, Drabik JR, Heikkila T, Bolson J, Sukop MC, Watkins DW, Rehage J, Mirchi A, Engel V, Letson D. Facilitating integration in interdisciplinary research: lessons from a South Florida water, sustainability, and climate project. Environ Manag. 2018;62:1025–37.
7. Wittenberg-Lyles EM, Oliver DP, Demiris G, et al. Assessing the nature and process of hospice interdisciplinary team meetings. J Hosp Palliat Nurs. 2007;9:17–21.
8. Yagura H, Miyai I, Suzuki T, et al. Patients with severe stroke benefit most by interdisciplinary rehabilitation team approach. Cerebrovasc Dis. 2005;20:258–63.
9. Hansen J, Hewitt M. PACE provides a sense of belonging for elders. Generations. 2012;36:37–43.
10. Mui AC. The program of all-inclusive Care for the Elderly (PACE): an innovative long-term care model in the United States. J Aging Soc Policy. 2001;13:53–67.

11. https://www.npaonline.org/pace-you/pacefinder-find-pace-program-your-neighborhood. Accessed 14 Jul 2020.
12. https://www.medicaid.gov/medicaid/long-term-services-supports/pace/programs-all-inclusive-care-elderly-benefits/index.html. Accessed 30 Jun 2020.
13. https://www.cms.gov/Regulations-and-Guidance/Guidance/Manuals/Downloads/pace111c08.pdf. Accessed 30 Jun 2020.
14. Nash M, Foidel S. Neurocognitive behavioral disorders: an interdisciplinary approach to patient-centered care. Cham: Springer; 2019.

Chapter 11
The Role of Social Work in PACE

Heather Hill and Janice Braxton

The aging of the U.S. population has brought about challenges and opportunities for older adults and their families. As a society, the need to adapt policies, programs, and resources to meet the needs of this complex, diverse, and expanding segment of our population has never been greater. The desire to understand the social, economic, political, and cultural consequences of growing older and address these consequences through creative care-delivery systems has created new areas of study and practice.

Gerontology is an area of specialization that focuses on the needs, problems, and opportunities that accompany people as they age [1]. As a field, gerontology is considered a multidisciplinary specialty that incorporates the perspectives of multiple disciplines to better understand the experience of what our society defines as old age. The specialty of gerontology includes physicians, nurses, educators, social workers, and others who seek to focus clinical care for our older adults through specialized medical care, community involvement, and advocacy efforts on both a personal and societal level.

Gerontological social workers understand the experience of aging and work to improve the lives of older adults and their families. Gerontological social workers are trained to understand an individual through the developmental life cycle by recognizing the unique developmental shifts and psychosocial needs that this population faces while transitioning into and through old age. Although many older adults face challenging life situations that may be exacerbated by losses of social support and declining functional and cognitive status, we can learn much through working

H. Hill (✉)
Social Work Department, Providence ElderPlace, Portland, OR, USA
e-mail: heather.hill@providence.org

J. Braxton
Social Work Department, Piedmont Health Senior Care, Burlington, NC, USA
e-mail: braxtonj@piedmonthealth.org

M. K. McNabney (ed.), *Community-Based Integrated Care for Older Adults*,
https://doi.org/10.1007/978-3-031-05137-1_11

with, observing, and learning from a population with a history of resilience and varied life experiences.

Social Workers and PACE

Social work is an integral discipline within the PACE model of care. Within the interdisciplinary team (IDT) of nine disciplines, the social worker stands within the clinical subgroup defined as the primary care team comprised of the primary care physician (PCP), registered nurse (RN), and social worker (MSW) (see "The Interdisciplinary Team and Process in PACE" chapter). The PCT works in alignment to provide overall medical and psychosocial care to all PACE participants.

Psychosocial Care

Social Workers (MSWs) provide psychosocial care by seeking to understand a person's medical needs in the context of his/her/their personal background, current social environment, and individual set of values. This "person in environment" model of understanding human behaviors and needs is just one of the unique ways in which the social work discipline adds value to the traditional medical team. Social workers educate and inform other members of the PACE IDT on the psychosocial aspects of a person's life that may be impacting health status, medical goals, well-being, and the ability to live safely in the community.

The PACE model of care and medical social work have long recognized the importance of whole-person care and how an individuals' environment and background directly impact health outcomes. Social Determinants of Health research is clear in demonstrating that programs which include social workers demonstrate improved cost-effectiveness and health outcomes [2].

Psychosocial Assessment

Upon enrolling in PACE, every participant receives a thorough psychosocial assessment. Social workers are uniquely positioned to identify a person's strengths and unique resiliencies. They also identify psychosocial barriers to medical care, such as behavioral health concerns, limited family and social support, language and health literacy issues, inadequate housing, food scarcity, and interpersonal abuse, neglect, and exploitation.

As such, PACE social workers consider how the following interrelated facets of an individual's life impacts overall medical needs and quality of life:

- *Social:* Family and support systems; housing, food and practical needs; culture and spirituality
- *Intrapsychic:* Personal values and identity, emotional and behavioral patterns, trauma history
- *Medical:* Understanding of medical conditions, health literacy, healthcare preferences

After assessment of the psychosocial needs of the participant, the social worker adds treatment goals to the overall PACE Interdisciplinary Team (IDT) care plan. Careplanning in PACE is a critical process that reflects the ongoing conversation between the PACE participant and the care team regarding treatment goals, values, and preferences (see "Care Plan" chapter). The PACE team members understand that participant-centered care depends on understanding the unique perspectives of the participant's own functioning and needs. Additionally, identifying and addressing the social determinants of health likely improves treatment compliance as well as emotional well-being [3].

Psychosocial Intervention

In addition to semi-annual assessments, PACE social workers provide ongoing care coordination and psychosocial interventions to support participants in actualizing their medical care goals through the continuum of care. **The scope of clinical practice for a medical social worker within PACE is wide-ranging. Interventions include providing linkages to appropriate community and environmental supports, facilitating family care conferences, empowering participants and caregivers to address complex medical and life decisions, enhancing coping skills to promote healthy behaviors as well as offering specialized palliative care and behavioral health support**.

Throughout social work practice, certain values inform all practice decisions and choices. Among these values, **personal autonomy and self-determination** are foundational in a social worker's practice and critically important in the provision of healthcare. Traditional models of healthcare can be challenging to navigate, and the participant's voice is not always heard or understood. In these traditional settings, it is often the responsibility of the medical social worker to bring understanding to issues related to patient autonomy, self-determination, and shared decision-making (with regard to care decisions and treatments) [4]. **The person-centered and autonomous philosophy of care that is embedded in social work practice directly aligns with the participant-centered model of care that defines PACE**.

Palliative Care

PACE provides medical and psychosocial care through the continuum of an individual's medical care needs, from enrollment through the end of life. Palliative care offers a perspective of care that focuses on values-based decision-making, medical and psychosocial symptom management, participant-centered care plans, and enhancing quality of life, as defined by the partcipant. By offering palliative care as an integrated service, the PACE primary care team (PCT) and IDT can maintain meaningful relationships with participants that reflect a deep understanding of their care needs and treatment preferences that lead to enhanced care through the end-of-life.

There is considerable overlap in the philosophy of social work and palliative care. Both advance the goals of bringing the participant perspective to IDT discussions and care planning. In conjunction with the PCP and RN, social workers skillfully facilitate participant and family understanding of health status, disease progression, and treatment goals. By partnering with participants and families, social workers advocate for proactive advance care planning to ensure that a health care representative has been identified and end-of-life decisions are well documented and reflect participant wishes. Social workers are trained to provide reflective, emotional support to PACE participants and their families through medical transitions and losses. Social work psychosocial interventions that focus on life review, anticipatory grief, and emotional symptom management are expected needs of participants faced with a life-limiting diagnosis.

Social Workers are a pivotal member of the team with regard to the care planning process, working collaboratively with participants to formulate treatment goals that focus on promoting psychosocial well-being and removing barriers to medical care. A participant's treatment goals are reflected in the initial care plan and revisited at least every 6 months for either continuation of current goals or modification based on changing psychosocial needs. Care planning and reassessment are opportunities for the IDT clinical disciplines to review and share participant goals to ensure cohesive alignment and coordination of care between members of the care team. Social Workers, as part of the primary care team, are required by PACE regulation to conduct clinical assessments and update care plans every six months to ensure responsive and medically appropriate psychosocial care.

Behavioral Health

Supporting a person's behavioral health is increasingly seen as a critical aspect of whole-person care within the PACE model. Historically, mental health and medical care at the primary care level outside of PACE have existed in silos; a person's mental health needs were addressed through referral to outside specialists. This approach of separating aspects of care defies the value of whole-person and well-coordinated care. The value of integrating behavioral health care within PACE medical clinics is taking hold. This integration model ensures more coordinated and comprehensive care for the well-being of our participant population [5].

Social workers are trained and licensed to provide both primary and specialty behavioral health services and are well positioned within the IDT to support the primary behavioral health care needs of PACE participants. As part of the initial and ongoing psychosocial assessment, the PACE IDT social worker identifies current and historical behavioral health concerns and then the primary care team (PCT) formulates a plan of care for the participant which may involve medication management, referral to a treatment or behavioral specialist, and/or working with the primary social worker to address normative grief, loss, interpersonal and transition issues.

Dementia

PACE programs, by nature of the population they serve, support a significant number of individuals with a diagnosis of dementia. Data indicate that the number of older adults who are developing dementia is increasing at a significant rate, with Alzheimer's disease listed as the fifth leading cause of death in people aged 65 and older [6]. The National PACE Association provides disease management recommendations through a PACE Dementia Model Practice tool that is adapted from evidence-based guidelines that are available to PACE programs [7].

These specialized interventions involve the entire IDT, providing wrap-around, comprehensive services to those most at-risk for psychosocial complications associated with dementia. Social workers play an important role in caring for participants and their caregivers by providing psychoeducation and support to family members and caregivers regarding the progression of dementia, caregiver strategies for managing communication and behavioral issues, and coping strategies to manage stress. This type of caregiver support is critical as the symptoms of dementia can be very challenging to caregivers, who are at risk of caregiver burnout. The stress of caregiving places a hardship on the family and the participant, threatening the well-being of all involved including the well being, safety, stability, and living situation of the participant.

Summary

The PACE model of care offers many opportunities for social workers to support participants in meaningful ways. Social workers partner with, and stand as advocates for, the participant by assessing and mitigating the psychosocial barriers to effective medical care. Equally valuable is the partnership with the other disciplines of the PACE interdisciplinary team to promote well-coordinated and effective care for disease and disability management in an effort to increase quality of life and enhance well-being for all those that we serve.

References

1. Sasser JR, Moody HR. Gerontology: the basics. New York, NY: Routledge; 2018.
2. Counsell SR, Callahan CM, Clark DO, et al. Geriatric care management for low-income seniors: a randomized control trial. JAMA. 2007;298:2623–33.
3. Craig S, Frankford R, Allan K, et al. Self-reported patient psychosocial needs in integrated primary health care: a role for social work in interdisciplinary teams. Soc Work Health Care. 2016;55:41–60.
4. National Association of Social Workers. NASW code of ethics; 2017. Available from https://www.socialworkers.org/About/Ethics/Code-of-Ethics/Code-of-Ethics-English
5. National Pace Association (NPA). Behavioral Health Operational resources Tool Kit; 2017. Available from https://www.npaonline.org/sites/default/files/2086_behavior_health_workbook_v6.pdf
6. Alzheimer's Association. Facts and figures; 2019. Available from https://alz.org/alzheimers-dementia/facts-figures
7. National Pace Association (NPA). Dementia Model Practice; 2014. Available from https://www.npaonline.org/

Chapter 12
The Role of Recreational Therapy in PACE

Susan Disman and Kelsey Ellis

Recreation Therapists (RTs) use participants' leisure interests to achieve goals and can help participants apply all skills they have learned in real life situations.

Recreational Therapy, also known as therapeutic recreation, is a systematic process that utilizes recreation and other activity-based interventions to address the assessed needs of individuals with illnesses and/or disabling conditions, as a means to psychological and physical health, recovery and well-being. Further, recreational therapy means a treatment service designed to restore, remediate and rehabilitate a person's level of functioning and independence in life activities, to promote health and wellness as well as reduce or eliminate the activity limitations and restrictions to participation in life situations caused by an illness or disabling condition [1].

This shift in healthcare demand combined with the fact that inpatient stays are getting shorter, highlights the need for community-based discharge sites where patients can continue their recovery and successfully reintegrate into the community. When individuals have a strong community-based setting to use after their discharge from the inpatient setting, the rate of re-hospitalization dramatically decreases and their overall health, recovery and quality of life improves. Their ability to actively contribute or give back to the community also improves [2].

S. Disman (✉) · K. Ellis
Providence ElderPlace Washington Providence St. Joseph Health, Seattle, WA, USA
e-mail: susan.disman@providence.org; kelsey.ellis@providence.org

M. K. McNabney (ed.), *Community-Based Integrated Care for Older Adults*,
https://doi.org/10.1007/978-3-031-05137-1_12

Benefits of Recreational Therapy in the PACE Model

Recreational Therapy is an integral part of a participant's treatment and lifestyle. Recreational Therapy can benefit participants by building confidence and self-esteem; improving physical abilities; decreasing isolation, loneliness and fear; strengthening interpersonal skills; managing stress; increasing quality of life; learning new skills and new approaches to old skills; developing new interests, and increasing social interaction. Get well, stay well, and live well [1, 3].

Assessment

Recreational Therapy services start with an assessment, which has several purposes. It gives the therapist a baseline of functioning and an idea of current and past leisure interests and identifies barriers to leisure involvement. Assessments are used to develop the plan of care, participant goals and group goals.

Initial Recreational Therapy assessments in the PACE setting have four core sections: current and past leisure interests, community involvement, barriers to leisure involvement, and analysis. RTs ask questions to reveal a participant's past and current leisure interests and investigate why they might not be participating in them. Are they physically unable to participate? Do they struggle with motivation or initiation? Do they have financial concerns? Are they unable to make a plan? Barriers to leisure include physical impairments, cognitive functioning, mental health diagnoses and cultural attitudes as well as leisure attitudes and skill sets. RT's also look at what social support a participant has to access their leisure. The RT looks at community involvement and access: what participants do in the community (i.e., shopping, going to the movies, place of worship, out to eat), how they function and how they travel in the community. After the evaluation is completed, RT analyzes the data to develop goals.

The reassessment process is similar to the initial assessment and is completed every 6 months. However, rather than looking at past leisure, RT's look at how the participant has changed since the last assessment. In the PACE setting, RT's look at leisure involvement, community access, community resources and leisure adaptations. They evaluate how a participant has changed in the past 6 months and what barriers to leisure the participant is encountering. In both the initial and reassessment process, the RT gathers information from the participant, family, friends, guardians and caregivers to build a well-rounded picture of the participant.

The Recreational Therapy assessment helps therapists develop an individual plan of care and build a day health program based on participants' needs and interests.

Care Planning Goals for Recreational Therapy

Like other members of the interdisciplinary team (IDT), RT creates a care plan for each participant based on information gathered in their assessments. In the PACE setting, these care plans are developed when a participant joins the program (initial) and every 6 months thereafter (reassessment).

Recreational Therapy care plan goals have a time frame and are measurable, attainable, and realistic. RT goals are created from information obtained during the assessment process. If a participant indicates they used to be "crafty" during the assessment, but they are not working on crafts anymore, this would cue the RT to evaluate why this change has happened. If a participant indicates difficulty initiating this activity, the RT would incorporate the participant's diagnosis of depression into the care planning process. The RT goal could be, "Over the next 6 months, participant will join arts and crafts class at assisted living facility (ALF) 1×/week." Interventions could include, "Review ALF activity calendar with participant, work with ALF activity staff and participant to attend weekly art class, check in with participant weekly to assess progress." If a participant indicates they are not working on their crafts due to decreased hand function, the RT would incorporate the participant's diagnosis of arthritis into the care planning process. The RT goal could state, "Over the next 6 months participant will use adaptive equipment to engage in one craft activity a week. Interventions would include work with participant to identify preferred craft activity, identify and obtain appropriate adaptive equipment, work with participant to successfully use equipment."

Participant Goals

Participant-driven goals are important. **At the end of the assessment, the RT will discuss what leisure-related goals the participant has identified for the next 6 months.** Setting their own leisure-related goal empowers participants to work toward their own objectives.

For example, a participant may mention the desire to go to the library, start knitting again, or learn to use a smartphone. Sometimes a participant identifies a goal that is unrealistic. The RT can help the participant examine the root of the goal and find a way to make that goal more realistic and achievable. When a participant identifies something they want to accomplish, the RT takes steps towards assisting the participant in achieving that goal. Participant goals are a key facet of the care plan and are incorporated into the discipline-specific goals and interventions.

Interventions

RTs develop and implement individual, evidence-based interventions. **RTs will use participants' leisure interests to accomplish their goals. One-to-one interventions vary by participant.** One common intervention is learning how to access the community independently. This could include using various transportation options, learning about community resources, and finding accessible and affordable leisure. Another intervention is learning how to reduce stress. This might include meditation, aromatherapy, relaxation, therapeutic coloring[4] and journaling. Other interventions include identifying ways to increase leisure participation, use of adaptive equipment, and incorporating behavior management. RTs work with participants, families, and caregivers to develop home leisure participation. For example, if a family member or caregiver expresses concern about a participant being bored or not doing anything, the RT will suggest leisure activities that match the participant's interests. The RT will then develop a plan with the family member or caregiver with specific steps to ensure progress towards the goal of being more active and engaged. If a participant's engagement in leisure is limited by a physical impairment, the RT will identify adaptations that will aid in participation of the leisure pursuit as independently as possible. For example, if a participant has hand tremors and their passion in life is fishing, the RT can adapt the fishing pole so the participant can be self-sufficient. The RT can also assist participants with setting up and using appropriate technology. This can include use of phones, tablets and computers, as well as downloading apps, and using adaptive technology. The RT can work with participants, families and caregivers to provide appropriate activities for participants living with dementia. The RT uses leisure education to help participants living with dementia identify activities that are meaningful and appropriate and will engage them with families and caregivers.

Putting It All Together

During an assessment, a participant living with Parkinson's disease identified a goal of "wanting to dance like Michael Jackson." The RT was able to assist the participant to achieve that goal by finding a free community Parkinson's dance class near the participant's bus line. The participant was hesitant to go to the class, but the RT arranged to go with her on the bus and stay with her throughout the class. Since this was part of her therapeutic treatment, the PACE program paid her bus fare. As a result of this advance planning and problem solving, the participant agreed to try the class with the help of the RT. On the day of the class, the RT met her at her home, and they walked to the bus stop together. The participant admitted to being nervous about the experience. The RT calmed her nerves by letting her know there would be ample rest times and she could always leave early. During class, they participated the entire time. After the class, the participant was more talkative, reminiscing on the bus ride home. A few weeks later the participant called the RT and reported that her tremors had subsided, and she felt more stable on her feet for the rest of the day after the class and asked the RT to accompany her to another class. The RT agreed to meet her at her class to encourage independence by taking public transportation. During the class, the participant was engaged and smiled throughout. When the class was finished, the participant reported she would continue this activity on her own. The RT was able to give the participant the tools and self-confidence to work toward a goal. This specific RT treatment plan increased her mobility, independence and confidence in the community and decreased symptoms from her Parkinson's disease that she experiences daily.

Recreational Therapist Role in the Day Health Center

The RT designs the day health center programs and works with the activity staff to implement programs, keeping in mind the participants' interests, needs, and function. Day health programs should be vibrant reflections of participant interests, cultural backgrounds and a place to create a community. Recreational Therapists design programs with activity group goals and participant goals in mind. Activities need to be challenging enough to keep the interest of participants but not so challenging that they want to give up. When needed, RTs provide adaptations to increase participation in day center activities. A day health program consists of general groups that all participants can attend as well as specialized therapeutic groups for a specific group of participants.

Recreational Therapy and General Activity Groups

General activity groups at a day health center are open to all participants**. RTs make sure that the calendar has a variety of activity groups in each domain, including cognitive, physical, emotional and sensory**. Cognitive activities can include crossword puzzles, mind games and lectures. Physical activities can include a variety of exercise classes, yoga, tai chi or bowling. Emotional activities can include spiritual care, creativity, relaxation and self-awareness. Sensory activities are designed to increase a participant's sensory awareness by stimulating the five senses (taste, smell, auditory, visual and tactile). In designing the day health program, RTs work with activity and day health staff to make sure the activity group content is age appropriate and challenging for all participants. RTs set up adaptations so everyone can participate in general groups. For example, if a participant has low vision and wants to attend the bingo group, the RT will enlarge the bingo card so the participant can read the letters and numbers independently. If a participant with a frozen shoulder wants to participate in the group exercise class, the RT will modify the arm exercises. The RT will then work with the activity staff to make sure they know and follow the modifications. RTs facilitate social interactions by introducing participants who have similar interests to develop a sense of community and friendship Activity staff are responsible to chart functional level on each participant in each group, usually in a flow-sheet format.

Recreational Therapy and Therapeutic Groups

A therapeutic group has defined goals for a specific group of participants and may be time-limited. The group itself has a goal and each individual participant has their own goal. There is a purpose to each group, which is targeted to individual participants. The RT will set clear expectations at the beginning of the group and talk to participants to set individual goals. One example of a therapeutic group is art journaling. Goals for the group could be to: start an art journal, learn art journaling techniques, work on their journals at home and bring them in once a week to process their work, or identify and express different feelings in their art journal. One participant's individual goal may be to identify a feeling (other than good, nice, fine, or happy); another participant's goal may be to successfully use an adaptation to grip a marker to create their art. RTs chart progress toward goals in their documentation. The RT evaluates the group, including where improvements can be made, progress toward each participant's goal, achievability of group objectives, and the necessary modifications or adaptations required for each individual.

What RTs Brings to the PACE IDT

Recreational Therapists are educated in the holistic approach to treating people, which fits perfectly with the PACE model. As a member of the IDT, the RT brings this outlook to every team meeting. The RT often observes participants in different settings than other clinicians. This gives the Recreational Therapist a unique viewpoint of the participant that is valued by the IDT. During IDT meetings, Recreational Therapists may report on functional changes with the participant. This could also include behavioral concerns at the day health program or at home, communication reports with caregivers and family members concerning leisure involvement at home, reports of boredom, safety concerns about leisure involvement, and changes in a participant's involvement in day health groups. When the Recreational Therapist receives a referral from another IDT member, they will report the outcome to the referring discipline and the IDT.

Summary

RT plays an integral role as a member of the IDT in a PACE setting. RT's not only use the recreational therapy assessment to develop goals of care, individual participant goals, and interventions, but they also integrate participant's leisure interests to achieve goals, develop the day health program, and facilitate individual treatments sessions. They approach every participant with a holistic mindset and work on developing their plan of care with the hopes of increasing each participant's quality of life.

References

1. Roberts S, Passmore T. Exploring contemporary therapeutic recreation services. NRPA; 2018. https://www.nrpa.org/parks-recreation-magazine/2018/october/exploring-contemporary-therapeutic-recreation-services/.
2. Flett JAM, Lie C, Riordan BC, et al. Sharpen your pencils: preliminary evidence that adult coloring reduces depressive symptoms and anxiety. Creat Res J. 2017;29:409–16.
3. American Therapeutic Recreation Association. About recreation therapy. https://www.atra-online.com/page/AboutRecTherapy. Accessed 24 Mar 2021.

Chapter 13
The Role of Transportation in PACE

E. J. Rice and Matthew K. McNabney

Transportation is defined as a mode of moving things and/or people from one place to another. Or even to take someone to another place in their mind with a strong emotion. PACE programs aspire to do both. In the general population of older adults, it is critically important to assist people getting to where they want to go with efficiency and skill.

There are two main "types" of transportation: *emergent and non-emergent*. When we consider **emergent** types, these are ambulances and air transit vehicles (helicopters and airplanes). For the vast majority of local/regional transports, traditional ambulances do the job for emergency needs. **Non-emergent** transportation is another layer of service that assists a large number of older adults on a regular basis with getting to and from necessary events. These include medical appointments and testing. An inability to access these transportation services can lead to lower quality medical care and social isolation.

Transportation for Older Adults in the General Population

Family and friends provide a great deal of transportation assistance to older adults in the community. This is critical to meeting the needs of daily life (shopping, medical appointments, social events). However, that can take a toll on those individuals and may become less reliable over time.

Public transit is an option but require familiarity with routes and schedules that can be overwhelming and sometimes unreliable. There can also be

E. J. Rice · M. K. McNabney (✉)
Hopkins ElderPlus, Johns Hopkins University, Baltimore, MD, USA
e-mail: erice11@jhmi.edu; mmcnabne@jhmi.edu

M. K. McNabney (ed.), *Community-Based Integrated Care for Older Adults*,
https://doi.org/10.1007/978-3-031-05137-1_13

problems with access to these services, even with recent changes to accommodate people with disabilities.

There are also "paratransit" services in many areas which offer rides (upon request) that operate during usual business hours and are designed to assist older adults with special needs. These require planning ahead (to schedule) and some flexibility due to the variability of ridership and the need to accommodate so many without the same destination (like the PACE center) or management that is not part of the same organization as the rider (like PACE).

Transportation in the Program of All-Inclusive Care for the Elderly (PACE)

We live in a society that seems to be in constant motion. Trying to get from one place to the other in the most efficient and safest way possible, not to mention comfortable. Our journey into the where with all of Hopkins ElderPlus (a PACE program) starts with and ends with our participants.

Our participants are the sustenance that moves HEP Transportation to higher standards in the conveyance industry. As they board our buses, they leave their sometimes-singular world to an intimate everyday all-day place that will love, cherish and take care of them for the remainder of the days we are together.

The objective in PACE transportation is to stimulate and move with efficiency and purpose, which is applicable to all the participants who make their way onto our vehicles. The care and concern that is shown by both the Driver and the Escort is part of our daily repetition.

Typical Day for PACE Transportation Team

7 am: The PACE transportation team members (drivers and escorts) arrive to the Team Conference Room for the daily briefing. This not only sets the expectations of the day, but also the tone and mood. All eight escorts are present and accounted for—with smiles not only on their faces but also in their temperaments. The eight drivers too, with their countenances glowing, assemble around the oblong conference table. They are ready for whatever road hazards and road rage they will encounter this day. Without hesitation and seemingly on cue "People, people, people" rings out from the baritone voice of the transportation coordinator.

His greeting is met with laughter and imitation. The day is off to a most ostentatious start as the theme of Hill Street Blues plays in the head of the coordinator as he begins the meeting. He hands out assignments to all in the room, answers the handful of questions and emphasizes the appointments. There are two main transportation objectives discussed. The routine but important task of getting participants to and from the day health center (DHC) for the "scheduled day" of social activities, rehabilitation, meeting with social workers and other staff, as well as medical care in the PACE clinic. There are also transportation requirements to get participants to outside appointments (those appointments away from the PACE campus). These are typically for tests or visits to medical specialists but can also be for personal business. There are also occasional and special "trips" sponsored by the PACE program to a movie or restaurant that requires the involvement and support of the transportation team.

The transportation coordinator also gives recognition during the morning meeting to the previous day's victories and responds to yesterday's opportunities. "We had a good day Friday. Thank you all for your efforts and accomplishments, all of the participants were delivered to their respective appointments and then back home without incident. This is the expectation for the everyday business of caring for and transporting our family, friends and loved ones." The coordinator finalizes the dialogue by requiring everyone to "Be Safe."

The drivers. Every PACE program has a staff of drivers to manage the vans and get the participants safely from here to there. This staff has a tremendous responsibility and must be carefully selected for this role. Examples of the requirements to the job of driver at one PACE program include:

- High school level of education
- Two years of previous driving experience
- Valid state driver's license with no more than 2 points prior to employment and no more than 3 points after employment (these must be verified)
- Adequate reading skills and ability to understand instructions, add/subtract numbers and make comparisons between numbers and letters
- Ability to exchange information on factual matters, schedule appointments, greet visitors, explain medical center policies, and/or relay messages to the appropriate personnel. This type of interaction requires courtesy and tact when dealing with patients, visitors and/or medical center employees
- Physical/mental/visual capabilities—stooping/bending, reaching/grasping objects, sitting for extended periods of time

Drivers must complete annual organization-wide safety and infection control updates, as well as annual department/unit-specific mandatory updates. There are also several established "service excellence standard" which are assessed by the coordinator (supervisor) on an annual basis.

The escorts. It is critical that PACE participants get to where they need to be *safely*. That not only requires highly competent and safety-conscious drivers to navigate the roads, but **there must also be attentive and well-trained staff (called "escorts") to address personal needs of participants during transit, to assist with boarding and exiting the vehicles and to address care needs during**

the ride. Escorts become very familiar with participants on their particular "runs" which greatly enhances the ability to positively impact the experience for the riders and increases the likelihood the issues will be properly interpreted and addressed.

The vehicles. Medical transport "vans" are standard vehicles for PACE programs. These are typically multi-passenger vans which have bench seats to accommodate those who can walk and be safely seated (with seatbelts) as well as space for those who require wheelchair support and can be "locked down" in the proper space on the vans. Smaller cars/SUVs are also used and offer more flexibility for smaller numbers of people or special circumstance, when appropriate. PACE program may also operate or maintain contracts with companies that provide ambulance transport services for situations when participants require more supervision or better ability to get someone in/out of a situation. There also must access to mechanic services to address maintenance as well as urgent repairs when needed.

7:35 am: The drivers leave the meeting to inspect their assigned vehicles, filling out the DVIR (Driver Vehicle Inspection Report). They then map or adjust their schedule to pick up the participant in the most efficient and cost-effective routes. For the most part, these routes and assignments are clustered geographically but exceptions keep the routine "flexible" for all drivers and escorts. The driver acts as the "second escort"; first driving and steering the van with no more than 14 passengers in the vehicle. The typical transport vans are capable of transporting up to four-wheel chairs at a time. This capacity does vary and must be considered in real time as decisions about deploying vehicles is made by the coordinator.

The escorts leave the morning meeting to call all participants on their assignment sheet. Reminding them and their loved ones that they are on the schedule to come to the DHC (Day Health Center) on that day. They also make the call to give them an estimated window for pickup time.

The mood on the vans is variable. There might well be singing and laughter but can often be a "quiet" ride with little chatter. However, the drivers and escorts typically try to create conversation and socialization. Changes in mood or willingness to converse are often the sign of another problem—possibly medical or psychosocial. This observation and subsequent report to the medical staff is key to the success of PACE management.

The driver and escort teams leave the morning meeting and head for the vans. At this particular PACE site, there are eight vans (each with one driver and one escort). A typical "run" will cover between 2–15 miles (round trip) and take up to 1 h, but this varies drastically due to PACE programs service area. Rural PACE programs can see much longer travel times. For any trip longer than 45 min (one way), it is required that the van stop and offer passengers a break and/or opportunity to use the toilet. As described before, the pick-up and drop-off is "through the door" service, as needed. Many times, participants and/or caregivers ensure readiness for curbside pickup, but this is often not the case.

On most days, there is the "second run"; the vans with the two staff members return the field for another round of passengers to travel to the PACE center. All told, there can be up to 2+ h for all of the people to be picked up and delivered to the center. The process reverses itself in the afternoon, starting at around 2 pm. These times vary based on size of the PACE program, size of service area and distance of trips.

The important roles of drivers and escorts go far beyond getting people from here to there. They are the **first to see them in the morning at pickup and the last to see them at the end for the day**. They recognize important changes from the last time we interacted with them that may very well go unnoticed by some staff members.

1. How is their speech?
2. Are they more irritable than the previous (or typical) day?
3. Are they able to ambulate with minimal discomfort?
4. How is their attitude?
5. How is their morning going so far?

Additional important messages to reinforce to participants: *we care about you, we want to do a good job for you, please let us know if you need anything or if any messages need to be passed along to other PACE staff members.*

2:30-3 pm—This is the time to round up of participants in the day health center (DHC), prepare to load the vans, maintain organization of the process (to avoid chaos), and to ensure that everyone gets safely on the vans. The participants return home by van with the same methods of observation and assistance as when picked up in the morning. The staff carefully note any changes from the morning to afternoon ride.

After drop-offs are completed, the vans are wiped down and swept out daily, preparing for the occupation of the participants. The vans are filled with fuel in the afternoon (after drop-off), to minimize the time a participant spends on the bus.

Challenges are met with excitement and expectations. A previous Transportation Supervisor encouraged his staff by reassuring his staff about the ever-changing landscape of the work… "That's what we do."

Participation in care planning process (ICP) by members of transportation team; report of how things are going for participant with transportation.

Some examples of the unique services of PACE transportation:

- Having heard that one PACE participant was being discharged from the ED after almost 36 h of evaluation, the transportation staff extends the time of service into the early evening to ensure that the participant is taken home by familiar faces after an exhausting experience.
- Realizing that a vanload of older participants (who happen to be nuns) enjoy singing, the driver and escort regularly join in for singing hymns and spirituals on the 35-minute drive back to the convent.
- Challenged by the physical barriers of Maryland rowhomes, the Hopkins ElderPlus transportation team acquired and mastered the operation of "scalamobils®"—stairclimbing devices which attach to wheelchairs and safely ascend and descend stairs.

Summary

As previously stated, getting people from here to there is only small portion of what the transportation staff does for the PACE participants. They ensure safety, take great pride in the service they provide and integrate fully into the goals and schedules of the IDT. Because PACE is a "center-based health program," it is essential that transportation services exist, but it is a calling to provide the level of compassion and attention to detail which is part of every day at all PACE programs.

Suggested Reading

1. www.aarp.org/caregiving/home-care/info-2020/transportation-services.html. Accessed 9 Feb 2022.
2. Center for Medicare and Medicaid Service (CMS). Medicaid Non-Emergent Medical Transportation Booklet for Providers, April 2016.

Chapter 14
The Role of Direct Care Providers in PACE

April Holmes and Renee Newmuis

Introduction

Aides who provide direct patient care to older adults with disability and chronic medical needs are a vital part of health delivery and is provided in a number of care settings. **When family and other "informal caregivers" are not available or no longer able to provide the needed assistance, paid staff are needed.** This can be in the community (and typically coordinated by the patient or family) or provided in communal living setting (such as assisted living or nursing home).

PACE programs provide care as needed to participants regardless of setting. This can include assistance in the PACE day health center (DHC), on the PACE vans during transport as well as in-home personal care. Regardless of setting, there are important considerations and procedures in providing this care and assistance.

The primary duties of direct care providers (sometimes called "personal care aides") are to assist people with bathing, dressing and using the bathroom; reposition patients who are not ambulatory; assist patients with transferring in and out of bed and with walking; serve meals and assistance with eating.

Home health aides (HHA) assist adults living at home with some form of disability or illness who have trouble caring for themselves, and they may be allowed to administer medicine or check vitals with direction from a health care professional. Personal care aides help people with everyday tasks and self-care, supporting them socially and emotionally to help them work and interact with others. Licensed practical and licensed vocational nurses (LPN/LVNs) work in hospitals, providing basic care to patients under the guidance of doctors and registered nurses, as well as performing various administrative duties.

A. Holmes · R. Newmuis (✉)
Hopkins ElderPlus, Baltimore, MD, USA

M. K. McNabney (ed.), *Community-Based Integrated Care for Older Adults*,
https://doi.org/10.1007/978-3-031-05137-1_14

Geriatric nursing assistants should be comfortable working with older adults and acting as a caregiver. Patience, good interpersonal and communication skills, and an ability to be a team player will help in enhancing the career as a geriatric nursing assistant.

There are different roles and types of training among direct care providers. The titles of these roles often overlap, and we will discuss in more detail below. It is important for a PACE program to understand the staffing needs of its participants. This will change as the census grows and managers are constantly reassessing needs and making hiring projections to fill the important roles of direct care providers.

Another important overarching role for all direct care providers is to **observe changes in participants over time and to report changes to other staff members.** This "early alert" of changes allows the PACE team to have an advance warning to intervene and provider early assessment and treatment. This cannot be over-emphasized and is one of the key advantages of the PACE model.

Direct care providers also have many opportunities to establish relationships with participants over time. Due to the sustained need for assistance over time (for many individuals), there are opportunities to learn more about each other's personal stories and create closer bonds. This can elevate the spirits of older adults enrolled in PACE over time and may lead to better health outcomes over time.

Direct Patient Care Providers: What's in a Name?

Direct care providers include health care workers identified in a number of ways, including certified nursing assistants (CNA), geriatric nursing assistants (GNA), medication technicians (MT) and other titles.

Geriatric Nursing Assistant (GNA) typically provide care to patients who are 65 and older, with elements of care that they normally can handle on their own. *Certified Nursing Assistant (CNA)* is someone who typically provides more of a companionship and assist with personal hygiene. *Medication Technician* (MT) are ones who normally work in assisted living setting or an Adult Daycare such as Hopkin's Elder Plus, or hospital but are typically only allowed to give medication in an assisted living environment.

Geriatric Nursing Assistant (GNA) and Certified Nursing Assistant (CNA)

Geriatric Nursing Assistants provide care to older patients by completing the following tasks: dressing patients, helping with bathing and hygiene, moving bedridden patients, accompanying them for doctor appointments, running errands, monitoring health condition, changing bed linens, and serving meals. Those interested in a Geriatric Nursing Assistant position should be able to highlight the following aptitudes in their resumes: nursing expertise, bedside manner, a caring personality, stamina, good communication skills, and reporting of observations. Most example resumes in the field include a high school diploma and personal care training.

CNAs, or certified nursing assistants, support patient care in healthcare facilities by interacting with patients and helping to prepare medical equipment. This position differs significantly from that of a registered nurse as CNAs are not licensed to perform many of the duties of RNs. However, CNAs do work with doctors, nurses, and patients to provide care during short- and long-term stays at healthcare facilities.

Within a healthcare facility, CNAs often have more direct patient contact than other professionals. A CNA may assist patients with everyday tasks such as bathing, eating, and dressing. They may also monitor and record patient vital signs to assist with diagnostic and recovery processes.

CNA Duties and Responsibilities

Assist Patients with Daily Tasks. CNAs **provide assistance to patients with everyday tasks.** This can include delivering patient meals to hospital or care facility rooms, helping patients to dress, use the restroom, or groom themselves. CNAs determine the best way to help their patients, checking if they need anything to keep them comfortable and healthy.

Assess and Record Patient Vital Signs. During intake and throughout a patient's stay, CNAs monitor and record the patient's **vital signs** using a variety of medical technologies. These primarily consist of checking the patient's pulse, breathing patterns, and blood pressure to determine whether they are within acceptable levels. Depending on the facility, a CNA may also be approved to draw a patient's blood for further testing.

Maintain Patient Rooms. **CNAs are responsible for cleaning and organizing patient and examination rooms**. This can include changing linens on a patient's bed, cleaning areas where fluids may have spilled, and ensuring that the patient and doctors have everything they need on hand at all times. For examination rooms, this may include restocking supplies, such as gloves, and following proper disposal methods for potentially hazardous materials.

Prepare and Clean Medical Equipment. In many healthcare facilities, CNAs prepare and clean medical equipment that doctors and nurses use for procedures and patient care. This can include specialized machinery and tools that are used throughout the facility. CNAs also maintain clean facilities, preventing infection by sterilizing equipment before and after use, maintaining use records, and ensuring that items are properly stored between uses.

Observe Patient Conditions and Behaviors. **CNAs work closely with patients every day, contributing to long- and short-term treatment by carefully observing patients' health and wellness from day to day**. These observations include overall patient health, recovery progress after a procedure, and reactions to treatment. Additionally, CNAs update patient records to reflect new information and report any changes or potential health issues to doctors and nurses.

Communicate with Patients and Care Providers. **Because CNAs spend a significant amount of time with patients, they frequently communicate with patients, doctors, and patient representatives**. These communications may fall under the Health Insurance Portability and Accountability Act (HIPAA), so CNAs need to follow procedures regarding patient confidentiality while maintaining a flow of helpful information between concerned parties.

Medication Technician

Medication technicians perform a number of functions to support medical staff and assist with the care of patients. These tasks include checking up on patients and listening to their concerns, updating medical records, and administering medication. Medication technicians typically work under the guidance of experienced nurses or medical staff on teams with other technicians and physicians. There may be a requirement to work unsociable hours with this job, depending on the employer. This position is well-suited to people who are compassionate, organized, work well as part of a team, and have excellent attention to detail.

Medication Technician Duties and Responsibilities

Medication technicians work for a variety of organizations, which can affect the duties they take on. Based on job listings we analyzed, a medication technician's duties typically involve:

Administer Patient Medication

Medication technicians administer the correct medications and dosages to patients on a daily basis. They may liaise with senior nurses or medical staff regarding any changes to a patient's condition or amendments to their required medication.

Perform Medical Check-Ups

Medication technicians perform regular patient check-ups to make sure their symptoms are not getting worse and to monitor the effects of medication. They report and resolve any adverse effects as quickly as possible for the well-being of the patient.

Update Patient Records

After taking note of any changes in the patient's condition, medication technicians update their medical records as required. They may also help obtain medical histories.

Report Patient Complaints to Senior Nurses

If patients have any concerns about their symptoms or complaints about how they're feeling, medication technicians listen to these complaints and report them to senior staff members so that they can be assessed.

General Considerations for Direct Patient Care Providers

Each role has the ability to work together that will help the team with caring of older adults. Formal training programs (GNA/CNA) help get a grasp on how to perform important everyday tasks, like how to change bed linen while the patient is in it, how to use a Hoyer or even how to use the sit-to-stand device. There is also need for ongoing "in-service" training to ensure that skills are maintained, and new skills are learned after hire. Along with possibly assisting grandparents or older family members or a nursing home resident. Going to school for all three job types can also assist in learning the proper way to assist with everyday ADL, giving medication and learning just to sit and be a listening ear that some may need.

Direct care in a homecare setting incorporates many of these direct care skills—by learning all three roles—staff can provide valuable service with feeding assistance, listening to participants "vent" (since some may have stories for days on top of days), or just simply washing their back and being a helping hand or even showing family members easier ways to do some of the services we provide. Being certified in all three skills (CNA, GNA, MT) helps in other ways by allowing visits to family members and being the professional sometimes allow staff to have to be the voice for them.

Many PACE participants need these types of services because that is how they get into the program. However, there are some participants who have different needs from the program. It is the responsibility of the interdisciplinary team (IDT) to determine the needs of each participant including the amount of direct care. For example, certain participants might need help with medical issues and not need assistance. However, there are many who need a great deal such as bathing, medication reminders, eating reminders or just simply assisting with everyday ADL. There is another category of participant who may need assistance with grocery shopping or to simply wash their back and they let the staff know they can do the rest themselves and are somewhat independent but not as much as the 10% of the enrollees. **Unfortunately, it is also a reality that direct care staff can be met**

with hostility, aggression, mistrust and even racism and violence. This can jeopardize the care provider-patient relationship when it is often the most needed. It is important to be supportive of staff and to hear the details of how there has been inappropriate behavior by the patient. If this persists, there should be clear communication to all patients and family caregivers that this will not be tolerated and reassignment of the staff member is in order.

Summary

PACE offers a well-balanced program that utilizes a variety of direct care providers to meet the goals of keeping older adults living in the community setting. This includes providing assistance in various settings to allow people to stay in the least restrictive environment. This care structure creates opportunities for valuable relationships to develop between caregivers and PACE participants.

Direct Care Position	Typical Roles in PACE	Common Site of Care in PACE
Certified Nursing Assistant (CNA)	Perform basic nursing tasks; check vital signs; communication with members of IDT	Day Health Center (DHC); escort/assistance while in transport
Geriatric Nursing Assistant (GNA)	Perform basic nursing tasks; special training and skills in the care of older adults; check vital signs; communication with members of IDT	Day Health Center (DHC); escort/assistance while in transport
Home Health Aide (HHA)	Assistance with daily care (ADL) in the home; supervision/safety; social support/conversation; communication with members of IDT	Home setting
Medication Technician (Med Tech)	Perform basic nursing tasks; check vital signs; administer medications; communication with members of IDT	Day Health Center (DHC); escort/assistance while in transport

Suggested Reading

1. Job Hero https://www.jobhero.com. Accessed on September 10, 2021.
2. Bercovitz A, Moss A, Sengupta M, Park-Lee E, Jones A, Harris-Kojetin LD. An overview of home health aides: United States 2007. Natl Health Stat Report. 2011;19:1–31.
3. Pennington K, Scott J, Magilvy K. The role of certified nursing assistants in nursing homes. J Nurs Adm. 2003;33:578–84.

Chapter 15
The Role of Nursing in PACE

Mary Austin and Suzanne Fortune

Nurses play a central role in the care of older adults. Training includes a broad view of health and disease including the impact of physical, psychosocial and environmental factors. It is common for nurses to deeply engage with patients to ensure understanding of disease process and management plans. Regarding the care of frail older adults with multiple chronic conditions, nurses serve on the front lines of care at nursing homes, rehabilitation centers and hospitals. They are also critical part of the workforce in the outpatient setting. This background and skill set make nurses well-suited to provide key clinical roles within integrated care models such as the Program of All-Inclusive Care for the Elderly (PACE).

PACE embodies the philosophy of holistic, person-centered care. Nurses are able to practice a range of skills within the PACE model of care that may not be available to them in other care settings. PACE allows nurses to build relationships with participants that evolve over time as they care for the whole person, body, mind, and spirit. Nurses focus on promoting the participant's highest level of functioning with a holistic approach to care which is the central component of PACE. Also, nursing practice is based on a core principle of interdisciplinary planning and intervention, which is a key PACE fundamental. **The nurse on the interdisciplinary team (IDT) therefore adds a professional framework that is well-aligned with providing care to the frail older adult in the PACE model**.

Nurses interact with participants and their families during times of wellness and during times of acute and chronic illness. Person-centered care is much more than

M. Austin (✉)
Senior Pathways LLC, Phoenixville, PA, USA
e-mail: maustin@srpathways.com

S. Fortune
Quality and Patient Safety, Ascension Living HOPE, Wichita, KS, USA
e-mail: suzanne.fortune@ascension.com

M. K. McNabney (ed.), *Community-Based Integrated Care for Older Adults*,
https://doi.org/10.1007/978-3-031-05137-1_15

administering medical care and treatments. It may mean calling participants the morning of a scheduled procedure or surgery to encourage or reassure them, checking in on participants who suddenly lose a spouse or family member, or running out to bring food back to a participant after learning during an after-hours home visit the participant had not had dinner. Serving participants from a range of backgrounds challenges nurses to find ways to best meet the needs of participants and provide care within their cultural contexts.

The PACE model offers nurses the opportunity to participate as vital members of the IDT providing wrap-around care and services to participants. **Registered nurses (RN) and licensed practical nurses (LPN) may choose to serve in case management, the clinic setting, home care or care plan coordination, quality, and supervisory positions**. PACE nurses thrive in the family-like atmosphere of the PACE organization where disciplines and associates function as a team to meet the care needs of those they serve. Together they celebrate the triumphs and mourn the losses supporting one another professionally as well as personally.

PACE serves frail older adults, thus creating a wide variety of PACE participants to care for in the community and long-term care settings. PACE facilities and service areas provide needed care and services to people from varying cultural and educational backgrounds, socioeconomic levels, and lifestyles. Some participants live with family and require assistance with care and services, other participants live alone needing less assistance in their everyday tasks but may lack opportunities to socialize.

Serving frail older adults is more than just ensuring their basic needs are met. Individuals enrolling in a PACE program may lack the necessary resources to live safely in the community and have difficulty securing adequate and safe housing. Some PACE participants have substance abuse issues (or substance abuse histories) that have significantly impacted their physical and mental health. Many also suffer from significant comorbidities that have not been consistently managed due to inadequate resources. Prior to enrollment in PACE, local emergency departments are commonly used as a form of "primary care." Many PACE participants have not had access to dental or vision care in years. Overall, most new PACE enrollees have not had the intense levels of care coordination and chronic disease management that are required to maintain their highest level of health and functioning. Nurses play a key role on the PACE IDT to provide the care participants need by bringing a conceptual framework that promotes their health, independence, and quality of life.

Registered Nurse (RN)

The role of the RN is a quite diverse within the PACE model and varies greatly from program to program. The RN may serve in dual roles, including clinic nurses and RN Case Managers in smaller PACE organizations (PO) where larger POs may opt to split the positions of clinic nurse and RN Case Manager. POs determine their needs based on the size of their service areas, the number of enrolled participants, and their overall participant age and health demographic. The PACE model allows for flexibility in its organizational structure and programs may therefore add nursing positions and roles that meet participant and regulatory requirements.

The PACE model is designed for participants to receive much of their care in the PACE Center. Participants are scheduled for acute or routine visits with their healthcare providers in the PACE clinic. Nurses working in the PACE clinic obtain vital signs, review current concerns, medications, conduct diabetic foot checks, administer medications and treatments, assist medical providers with procedures, provide education, and a variety of other care as ordered. It is not uncommon for PACE sites to also employ triage nurses who assess participants with medical concerns while in the PACE Day Health Center, consult with other nurses and providers, and carry out medical provider orders for a variety of lab tests and procedures.

RNs also often serve in comprehensive roles providing "case management" type care to participants. The RN Case (RN) serving on the IDT oversees the care of an assigned group of participants. This team approach helps participants and team members develop and build trusting relationships that go a long way in earlier recognition of health and safety concerns that can result in fewer emergency department visits and hospitalizations. This team approach assists the IDT disciplines in identifying changes which can impact a participant's ability to continue living safely and independently in the community. From enrollment through the end of life, RNs often serve as the medical liaison between participants and other IDT disciplines. The RN's perspective and holistic approach contributes to the IDT process and often lends itself to promoting the overall management of the participant's plan of care.

Beginning with enrollment, initial assessments provide the foundation for building person-centered plans of care for PACE participants. RNs collect information about the participants' overall health, past medical and surgical histories, mental health concerns, family and caregiver support systems, and make recommendations for services to enable participants to live safely in the community for as long as possible. **Medication management is a core assessment of the RN to ensure participants are able to manage their medications safely, understanding when and how medications are to be taken, their common side effects, and the ability to self-administer**. RNs recommend methods of medication management for participants who may have difficulty safely managing their medications. These interventions may include the use of medications reminder calls, co-mingled packages, pill minders, and electronic medications boxes with alarms. After initial assessments, semi-annual assessments are conducted to assist the IDT to identify changes that may signal the need for revising participant goals and interventions, initiating new services or revising those already in place. Between semi-annual assessments, other assessments may be conducted when significant changes occur in caregiver support systems, biopsychosocial wellness, or when requests for services are voiced by participants, caregivers, or active participant representatives. Each assessment is equally important and presented to the IDT for discussion and determination, as are the assessment findings and recommendations of each discipline.

PACE RNs enjoy more autonomy than in other types of nursing environments. RNs set their schedules to see PACE participants in the PACE facility and the community, whether in participant homes or contracted long-term care facilities. PACE programs retain the responsibility for managing participant care across the continuum. Therefore, RNs may routinely visit contracted long-term care facilities to ensure participants are receiving needed care and services, visit with the facility nurses regarding participant concerns, and ensure facilities have the most current orders in participant charts. PACE RNs also provide care in participants' homes. However, as one PACE nurse described it, nursing in the traditional home health agency is often driven by insurance companies and reimbursement guidelines and is highly restricted in scope and flexibility. Obtaining needed resources is not always easy. However, in PACE model of care, PACE is the insurance company and can supply its nurses with the tools and supports needed to successfully manage their participants' health concerns freeing up time to spend with participants.

PACE is designed to provide care and services to participants from enrollment until death. In many ways, PACE organizations provide end of life care similar to a Hospice provider when participants are nearing the end of life, whether participants choose to die in the home or a facility. Ideally, end-of-life planning is begun before a participant is end stage. Along with the medical provider, the RN is often in the perfect position to prompt and facilitate conversations about end-of-life preferences. Because of the trusting relationships built with participants and their families, these issues often surface during assessments and following significant declines in health. RN Case Managers can be the liaison between the participant, their family, and the rest of the care team during end-of-life care, continually assessing, monitoring, and providing care and support until a participant's life ends. Not all nurses come to PACE with end-of-life care experience, and yet many find end-of-life care the most rewarding part of the care and services provided to participants and families.

PACE services include after-hours on-call services for participants experiencing acute care needs. Each PACE organization sets up their on-call services to best meet the needs of their participants and associates. RNs may rotate on-call duties, or the PO may choose to employ nurses for after-hours on-call duty only. Depending on the program, a medical provider and a nurse may be on-call after hours. Some POs utilize answering services to field calls to nurses or providers, while others may choose to provide participants with designated on-call numbers for providers and nurses. However POs opt to handle their after-hours on-call services, the RN is available to answer participant questions regarding medications, or medications deliveries, communicate with on-call providers, and may make home visits as needed to assess acute concerns and report assessment findings to the on-call provider.

Home Care Coordinator

The PACE Home Care Coordinator (HCC) is a vital member of the PACE IDT. A nurse most often fills this role. The HCC primarily assesses, recommends and oversees the services provided to participants in their homes (see Chap. 16). During the enrollment process, the HCC evaluates participant safety in the home environment. They may visit the homes of prospective PACE participants to obtain home safety information to share during intake coordination meetings. This alerts other IDT disciplines of concerns that may impact the POs ability to safely maintain participants in the community. Home Care Coordinators recommend home-care services to include assistance with Activities of Daily Living (ADLs), personal hygiene, dressing, eating, mobility and maintaining continence, and Instrumental Activities of Daily Living (IADLs), to include meal preparation, grocery shopping, transportation, laundry, housework, and communication availability and use. As participants' levels of function change as part of the natural aging process, illness, hospitalizations, or declines due to chronic illness, the Home Care Coordinator will make recommendations to the IDT to modify, increase, or decrease services in place, or recommend assessments by rehab therapists for potentially needed durable medical equipment (DME) to maintain participant safety in the home. When participants move within the community, the Home Care Coordinator conducts home safety assessments and reports findings and recommendations to the IDT.

This HCC role often interacts and collaborates with Occupational and Physical Therapists to decide on adaptive equipment and mobility devices best suited for the participant. The HCC also communicates with the home health aide (HHA) regarding individual needs and preferences of the participant. Equally important, the HCC can be the liaison between the HHA and the IDT regarding the participant's status, issues, and overall functioning. Since so much care is provided in the PACE center, the input and perspective of the HCC is important to rounding out the overall understanding of the participant's needs.

Licensed Practical Nurse (LPN)

Licensed Practical Nurses may hold positions within the PACE model of care. LPNs assist RNs in collecting ordered specimens, administering medications and injections, testing blood sugars, and various other activities as allowed under state laws.

The PACE clinic routine is often hectic and unpredictable, especially during key times of the day. The LPN often takes on a coordination role ensuring the flow of participants for routine and acute needs. They will also perform a variety of procedures such as lab draws, wound care, and respiratory treatments. LPNs can play a vital role in participants' medication management. They coordinate with the primary care providers to ensure medications are ordered and re-ordered on a timely basis and that medications are obtained by the participants. The LPN often administers medications to participants who require them during center attendance.

Nursing Assistants

Various positions in PACE are filled by nursing assistants or individuals with similar training (see Chap. 14). These staff are a critical part of the IDT and are included in the regulatory requirements that govern PACE to be a member of the IDT.

These staff members function as personal care attendants in the PACE Center, as home care assistants, and clinic staff. They play a very important role and often provide critical information to the IDT since they work so closely with participants on a day-to-day basis. It is often the nursing assistant that notices the early signs of acute illness, such as an unsteady gait or increased confusion. They form close relationships with participants and families who will often express to them their concerns sooner than they would to another IDT member. Nursing assistants utilize a variety of hands-on and communication skills on a daily basis to assist with meeting participants' needs.

PACE Administrative Positions

Nurses occupy essential key administrative positions at all levels in PACE organizations. **Since the success of PACE is based on highly effective management of the healthcare needs of a very complicated and frail population, the professional nurse is well-equipped to fill many key positions.** At the PACE center level, the Director of Clinical Services, Site Director, Quality Director, Education Coordinator, and Day Center Manager are usually RNs. Nurses often lead the Quality, Infection Control, and Education Departments. Leadership at the organizational level is often comprised of nurses including corporate executives (CEO, COO, VPs) and directors.

Summary

The PACE model of care provides opportunities for nurses to expand their skill set, operate as equal members of a team of professionals serving frail older adults and improving the quality of life for participants and families. It is not without its challenges, however. PACE participants become like family, making it difficult to watch as participants choose to ignore the recommendations to improve their health and wellness thereby causing themselves more suffering. As participants near the end of life, it is difficult to say goodbye. Yet, nurses who choose PACE as a career love their jobs and look forward to coming to work. The varied opportunities and family-like atmosphere allows nurses to embody the legacy of Florence Nightingale to minister to the poor and suffering.

"Nursing is more than just taking care of a person's body. Sometimes nursing is holding a family member's hand while their loved one dies. Sometimes it is coming up with ideas to help someone in the community remain there because they want to be independent, but struggle. Sometimes it is having those frank, oftentimes hard, conversations with people that may make them mad, but they need to hear." Sandy Carter, BSN, RN Ascension Living HOPE.

Suggested Reading

1. 42 CFR §460 Programs Of All-inclusive Care For The Elderly (pace) - Code of Federal Regulations (ecfr.io).

Chapter 16
The Role of Home Care in PACE

Anita Pope

General Overview of Home Care

Until the late nineteenth century, care for the sick and elderly was provided primarily by family members in the home. Doctors and hospitals were accessed as a last resort for severe illnesses that could no longer be treated with home remedies, and the aged generally lived out their lives in their homes while receiving care from family members, friends, and neighbors. Early home care organizations focused on maternal-child care and the ill and dying. These organizations were generally funded by donations from philanthropists; but in 1909, the Metropolitan Life Insurance Company (MLI) created a home care nursing benefit for their subscribers, believing that it would stimulate business by attracting new policyholders. Metropolitan Life policyholders received more than one million home care visits in 1916 through this benefit [1].

As the U.S. population aged and became chronically ill with longer life spans, it became evident through insurance claim data that home nursing and hospital services were more frequently utilized to support chronically ill patients. Activities of daily living (ADLs) made up the bulk of care provided by both services, which became a financial drain on insurance companies. To help finance care services for the elderly, Social Security was created in 1935 [1]. This allowed for the establishment of some private nursing homes for patients whose families were unable to maintain appropriate care in the home. Over the next two decades, the sheer volume of the elderly and chronically ill population overwhelmed hospitals and home care services across the country. Insurance companies began limiting home care benefits to the care of short-term illnesses with the expectation that the policyholder would recover and return to work, while the elderly and chronically ill were left to be cared for by family members or to be moved into long term nursing homes.

A. Pope (✉)
Rocky Mountain PACE, Colorado Springs, CO, USA

M. K. McNabney (ed.), *Community-Based Integrated Care for Older Adults*,
https://doi.org/10.1007/978-3-031-05137-1_16

Home care services were finally available to a broader population of patients when they were included in the Older Americans Act of 1965. Additional services provided to the aged population by Medicare were Meals on Wheels, elder abuse programs, and transportation services. Home care services under Medicare were provided according to medical necessity guidelines and were limited to intermittent episodes of care for acutely ill and homebound patients. Again, these services did not meet the ADL needs of aged or chronically ill patients but focused on skilled nursing services such as skilled nursing assessments, medication management and administration, and wound care. Some states provide long-term home care services under Medicaid for people with disabilities who require assistance with ADLs several times a day to remain independent in their own homes; in addition, Home and Community Based Services (HCBS) and In Home Support Services (IHSS) programs under Medicaid allow family members to be paid for providing home care services to their loved ones in certain states.

Home Care services under Medicare, Medicaid, and Medicaid waiver programs are subject to their own specific rules and regulations, and Home Care agencies are paid for their services by a traditional fee-for-service claims process.

Home Care and the PACE Model

PACE programs have their own set of regulations in the Code of Federal Regulations Part 460. These regulations cover all the services provided by a PACE program, which include all Medicare-covered items and services and establishes the PACE Interdisciplinary Team (IDT), which consists of eleven disciplines: primary care physician, registered nurse, master's level social worker, physical therapist, occupational therapist, recreational therapist, dietician, PACE center manager, home care coordinator, personal care attendant, and transportation [2]. The IDT meets regularly to establish, review, and revise the interdisciplinary care plan with the PACE participant and/or his or her representative. The PACE model of care incorporates social, wellness, support, and medical services to seniors with chronic care needs and their families in their community. Home care services play a large role in the overall care delivered by the PACE organization.

The exchange of information between the home care worker and the IDT is vital to providing real-time interventions to care needs for the PACE participant. Home care workers, including the RN, LPN, CNA, and PCW communicate their findings to the IDT on a regular basis, which helps the IDT to coordinate care. A reported change in condition generates a required assessment and interim care plan to address the identified need. For example, a CNA may observe during a home care visit that a participant is having difficulty rising from his chair; the CNA notifies the IDT, which then assigns a physical therapist to assess the participant's condition. The therapist brings her assessment back to the IDT and recommends a course of treatment or equipment, which is implemented by the appropriate discipline. The IDT updates the participant's care plan and evaluates the success of the intervention at the next care plan review.

Specific PACE Home Care Services

The provision of home care services by the PACE program is an essential part of the all-inclusive care model. Home Care staff are the eyes and ears of the IDT in the home; by interacting on a personal level with the participant in his or her living space, home care staff are able to collect and relay valuable data to the IDT for identifying changes in participant condition or unmet needs. Home Care services are provided in a variety of different ways, depending on the practices of the individual PACE program. Some PACE programs contract their home care needs out to home care agencies in the community; some PACE programs utilize clinic staff to provide home care services, while others establish a separate Home Care department within the PACE organization to provide these services [3]. PACE Home Care services are regulated differently than traditional Medicare or Medicaid home care services and allow for more interdisciplinary care management to ensure that all care needs are being met. The main goals of the provision of home care services by a PACE organization are to keep PACE participants as independent as possible in their current living situation, to provide person-centered care, and to decrease inappropriate emergency department visits by providing services for non-life-threatening medical issues in the home.

Contracting Home Care services through a community Home Care agency ensures that the burden of scheduling, staffing, and meeting State and Federal Home Care regulations lies with the contracted agency. In this scenario, the PACE organization would provide a referral to the Home Care agency for the required services and act as the insurance company for the PACE participant by paying for Home Care services rendered, according to the terms of the contract. The Home Care agency would be responsible for hiring and providing appropriate staff, verifying their discipline-specific competencies, staff payroll, and successfully passing all State and Federal regulatory surveys. The PACE organization is responsible for the upkeep of the referral and payment system to ensure that the Home Care agency is reimbursed for all services provided to PACE participants. The PACE organization is also responsible for monitoring the contracted Home Care agency for compliance with the contract agreement and corrective action plan for any deficiency that is identified.

Providing Home Care services through the PACE team involves the coordination of participant care needs and the assignment of visits by the provider, Care Coordinator, or other designated PACE staff. In some PACE organizations, participants receive part of their care in the clinic and part of their care at home; for instance, wound care might be provided once per week in the clinic during the regularly scheduled day at the center, with the remainder of wound care visits being provided in the home. Care in the home in this scenario is seen as an extension of clinic services to the PACE participant and is an especially convenient process for a newly established or small PACE organization with a small participant census. Under this model, nursing, nurse aide, and personal care worker staff are more fluid and move from the clinic to the home as directed (Table 16.1).

Table 16.1 PACE home care services

Nursing	Certified nurse's aide (skilled care)	Personal care worker (non-skilled care)
• Regulatory assessments • Care planning • Physical assessment • Wound Care • Medication administration • Teaching (medications, procedures, fall prevention) • Post-hospital follow-up • Post-ED follow up • Post-fall follow up • Same day triage	• Bathing • Dressing • Transfers • Toileting • Light housekeeping • Skin care • Grooming	• Bathing • Dressing • Toileting • Skin care • Grooming • Light housekeeping • Grocery shopping

Permission was granted by authors who created this table

Home Care Staff Considerations

The Home Care worker is an autonomous provider who spends most of his or her time in the community in participants' homes. Different communities, neighborhoods, and participant homes pose a diverse range of safety concerns, and the home care worker must be supplied with training and equipment to help maintain a safe working environment. One safety issue that home care workers frequently face in the home are pets, especially dogs; in this situation, the Interdisciplinary Team, Social Worker, or PACE Manager can ensure a safe environment for the caregiver by reaching an agreement with the participant to keep animals secured during home care visits. Another safety concern that home care workers may find in the home is the presence of cigarette smoking, smoking by the participant while wearing oxygen, and participant consumption of drugs or alcohol during the home visit. The PACE organization must supply workers with guidelines for addressing these concerns with the participant and must give them the ability to end the visit if necessary. Home care workers may also be exposed to inappropriate behavior by the participant, a friend, or family member in the home. The worker should be trained to handle this type of situation by de-escalation or by leaving the home and reporting the situation to their supervisor.

Outside of the participant home, the home care worker is faced with a variety of safety issues as well. Home care workers are required to complete visits during early morning and late evening hours, when lighting can be an issue; workers may be faced with car problems, such as flat tires; a motor vehicle accident may happen during travel between visits; or a home care worker may be required to perform care visits in a dangerous neighborhood. Safety training must be provided by the PACE organization to ensure that home care workers observe the best safety practices when out in the community.

Larger PACE organizations may find it more efficient to establish a Home Care department and staff it with dedicated nurses, nurse aides, and personal care workers to provide Home Care services. This scenario allows the organization to have more control over the staffing and scheduling of Home Care visits, and to streamline communication between the Home Care disciplines and the Interdisciplinary Team for the purpose of care planning and meeting the participant's overall health care needs. As PACE regulations mandate access to medical services 24 h per day/7 days per week, this need can be achieved by a dedicated Internal PACE Home Care department staff. Establishing a dedicated Home Care department also eliminates the need for contracting an outside Home Care agency and the manpower required for the upkeep of the flow of communication, billing, and payment for services required by a contracted agency.

The services that are provided by PACE organizations, whether by PACE Clinic staff, contracted community agency, or PACE Home Care department, are largely the same as those offered by typical community Home Care agencies; these include skilled and unskilled activities of daily living (ADLs) such as bathing, dressing, and assistance with mobility, and instrumental activities of daily living (IADLs) such as meal preparation, grocery shopping, and light housekeeping. Home Care services also include skilled nursing services, such as wound care, medication administration and management, regular periodic nursing and home care coordinator assessments, and nursing education for medication changes and upcoming procedures.

Physical, occupational, and speech therapy are also part of the PACE services that may be provided in the home setting as part of the Home Care plan or by a combination of in-center and in-home appointments. In addition, telehealth services may be added to the plan of care to augment or substitute for certain home care services when appropriate.

PACE Home Care and the Interdisciplinary Team

Ongoing and thorough communication is required between all the disciplines in PACE and the IDT for providing safe and efficient care. The IDT is responsible for coordinating the plan of care for each PACE participant [4]. The care plan spans a period of 6 months, according to PACE regulations, and is updated as needed when there is a change in the participant's condition. The IDT also tracks upcoming medical procedures, surgeries, and transfer from one level of care to another, so that appropriate interventions may be incorporated into the plan of care. Home Care Coordinators, a required member of the IDT, are responsible for functions such as scheduling and tracking home care appointments and regulatory assessments, triaging acute care needs, assigning staff to address those needs, and maintaining a current and complete plan of care. Observations from Home Care staff are disseminated to the IDT by the Care Coordinator, so that interventions may be initiated to address any needs that are not currently being met. These might include changes in the condition of the participant, equipment, supply, or food needs, or any housing or family needs that might require an intervention from the PACE organization. Continuity of care is also dependent upon the coordination between disciplines and between members of the same discipline.

Differences in PACE and Traditional Home Care

The direct care services that are provided in the home by a PACE organization or a traditional Home Care agency are basically the same: nursing services such as wound care, medication management, post-event follow up, and teaching, as well as assistance with activities of daily living provided by Certified Nurse's Aides or Personal Care Workers. Some differences in care delivery include the layering of care services rather than the discontinuation of one service to add another; for example, a PACE organization will layer PACE-provided home care services with Assisted Living services and Hospice services, rather than discharging the participant from Home Care to access Hospice services. Within a PACE organization, if a participant moves from an independent living situation to an assisted living facility (ALF), PACE Home Care will continue to follow the participant and provide care in addition to the services provided by the ALF.

Another difference in the two entities is mainly how each is regulated and reimbursed. Traditional Home Care services are regulated by Centers for Medicare and Medicaid (CMS) and each individual state regulatory agency. In a traditional Home Care agency, a patient who is covered by Medicare is expected to receive short-term services that are focused on recovery after an event, such as an injury or surgery. The care often involves physical or occupational therapy and short-term assistance with activities of daily living. The goal is to get the patient as close to their baseline functioning as quickly as possible, then to discharge them from the services. A Medicaid-covered patient typically receives home care services to maintain their baseline condition due to a chronic illness or disability. These services are generally long-term and focus on maintaining wellness and independence of the patient. Traditional Home Care agencies under Medicare and Medicaid must fulfill the requirement of documenting and submitting the Outcome and Assessment Information Set (OASIS) to CMS upon admission, discharge, and any change of condition between those two points in time. The OASIS contains data points that are related to reimbursement through Medicare and Medicaid.

In a PACE program, Home Care services focus on both the short-term and long-term needs, with the ability to move fluidly between the two. The PACE organization is also able to provide services that are generally not provided under Medicare and Medicaid, such as wellness checks and supply deliveries. Since PACE has its own regulations under CMS, the organization is not bound to the OASIS documentation and submission requirement; rather, PACE organizations use PACE-specific electronic health records (EHR), and care data is submitted to CMS through the reporting module of the EHR. Reimbursement for Home Care services is provided in the overall PACE program reimbursement and in managed care reimbursement, rather than fee-for-service.

Summary

The PACE organization strives to provide truly all-inclusive care, including Home Care services, to its participants. The program facilitates a high level of collaborative care between the members of the interdisciplinary team to prevent gaps in the health care continuum. The interdisciplinary nature of the PACE program allows for more interaction between disciplines, and the ability to create and maintain a long-term interdisciplinary care plan. Home Care services under PACE are subject to PACE regulations under CMS, which differ from traditional home care regulations in that the length of service is not limited and data submissions for reimbursement are specific to PACE. The PACE organization is able to keep participants on long-term Home Care services and also provide one-off visits when needed to those who do not require long-term Home Care. PACE Home Care workers are often the first team members to identify a change in condition due to close contact with participants in their homes, which facilitates an interdisciplinary care plan revision to meet the needs of the participant in any domain that is affected by the change.

Safety awareness and respect for the participant and his or her home are always important aspects of any home care service. The organization must be responsible for providing a safe care environment for both the participant and the Home Care worker. Services must be provided in such a manner that the participant retains his or her privacy and dignity.

Finally, the most important aspect of providing Home Care services in the PACE organization is communication between the participant, care coordinators, nurses and other Home Care workers, and the interdisciplinary team. When communication between the team members is thorough and timely, care of the PACE participant is facilitated more efficiently and effectively.

References

1. Buhler-Wilkerson K. No place like home: a history of Nursing and home care in the US. Home Healthc Now. 2012;30:446–52.
2. Office of the Federal Register. Code of federal regulations. Title 42, Parts 430 to 481; 2017.
3. National PACE Association. PACEFinder: Find a PACE program in your neighborhood. 2020. Retrieved from https://www.npaonline.org/pace-you/pacefinder-find-pace-program-your-neighborhood#:~:text=Currently%2C%20133%20PACE%20programs%20operate,click%20on%20your%20state%20below.
4. Centers for Medicare and Medicaid Services. Program of all-inclusive care for the elderly (PACE). 2020. Retrieved from https://www.cms.gov/Medicare-Medicaid-Coordination/Medicare-and-Medicaid-Coordination/Medicare-Medicaid-Coordination-Office/PACE/PACE.

Chapter 17
The Role of Medical Providers in PACE

Peter DeGolia, Gwen Graddy, and Matthew K. McNabney

General Medical Providers (Non-PACE)

Many medical providers who care for older adults in the community restrict their practice to ambulatory practice and are considered "primary care providers" (PCPs). There are also hospital-based clinicians ("hospitalists") who care for patients admitted to the hospital. This trend has led to discontinuity among providers and more confusion for patients. For example, decision-making for important decisions that are in response to hospital events are left to the hospital-based team that likely has no history with the patient prior to the admission.

Some PCPs do provide care in nursing homes, but many do not. That is also when patients experience discontinuity of care at a critical time. Whether for a short-term ("subacute" or skilled nursing home care) or long-term indication, older adults are vulnerable to changes in providers.

Similarly, very few (approximately 1.5%) providers make house calls and have a difficult time continuing to provide primary care to homebound patients. This also presents important challenges as health declines and care decisions are needed but difficult for most providers and their patients in this situation.

P. DeGolia
McGregor PACE, Cleveland, OH, USA
e-mail: peter.degolia@mcgregorctr.org

G. Graddy
PACE Southeast Michigan, Detroit, MI, USA
e-mail: Dr.Graddy@pacesemi.org

M. K. McNabney (✉)
Hopkins ElderPlus, Johns Hopkins University, Baltimore, MD, USA
e-mail: mmcnabne@jhmi.edu

M. K. McNabney (ed.), *Community-Based Integrated Care for Older Adults*,
https://doi.org/10.1007/978-3-031-05137-1_17

General Medical Providers in PACE Model

In the PACE model, medical providers remain involved in care regardless of care setting. The PACE model of care is primary care-based and biopsychosocial in orientation. The focus of medical services within PACE, different than a typical community-based primary care practice with limited social services, is to treat the whole person within the context of their community. The federal rules governing medical services in the PACE program require semi-annual comprehensive evaluations performed by the PCP. In addition to comprehensive, coordinated primary care, care coordination across the care continuum by the medical providers is very important. The model (and regulations) require that PACE programs (and the PACE PCP) remain involve during hospitalization—this includes authorization for the admission, communication and coordination of continued need for hospital care, and planning for discharge and any transition of care needs (nursing home care, home care, medication reconciliation). During and after inpatient stays, the PACE medical provider plays an important role in reducing 30-day readmissions. This is effectively done by helping coordinate the transitions of care by getting participants seen in a timely manner post-hospitalization, either at home or in the clinic. In addition, the PACE medical provider can help minimize the need for post-hospital nursing home admissions by leveraging the resources that PACE can provide both in the community and at the PACE center. The financing model (full risk/capitation) also creates a financial incentive to ensure the most efficient use of hospital-level care and to minimize the risk for readmission to hospital after discharge.

Therefore, PACE medical providers (particularly the medical director) remain engaged in care decisions across the continuum. Medical providers are also responsible for communicating medical events to the rest of the IDT. This communication is critical to the successful operation of the PACE team. There are vast resources within PACE (home care, social work, rehab) that can supplement medical care for PACE participants that experience illness. However, that requires clear and timely communication from the medical providers.

Types of Providers

Physicians (M.D., D.O.) are certainly important members of the PACE medical staff. Physicians are typically trained in the "primary care specialties" (internal medicine, family medicine) and some have additional training in geriatric medicine and/or palliative medicine. Rarely, physicians will be trained in another subspecialty of internal medicine. Regardless of training background, there is definitely a "primary care" mindset among PACE physicians.

Certified, registered nurse practitioners (CRNP) *and Physician Assistants* (PA) are important primary care providers in PACE. Serving the "PCP" role for PACE participants, CRNPs and PAs collaborate with physicians and also communicate directly with the IDT to coordinate care for large panels of participants. PACE regulations stipulate that CRNPs and PAs operate in similar manner to physicians with regard to fulfilling clinical roles within the IDT and in primary care.

Important PACE Roles for Medical Providers

Comprehensive Coordinated Primary Care

PACE primary care providers are engaged in all aspects of the health and well-being of their participants. Not only do they provide evaluation and management of medical problems, but they also work closely with other health care professionals within PACE to bring care and services to their participants to achieve the highest practical level of function. They work closely with the PACE Clinical Pharmacist to review and address medication management, striving to minimize unnecessary medications and monitor for potentially detrimental adverse effects. The PCP often works collaboratively with the PACE social worker to ensure safe and adequate housing for their participants. The PACE model of care enables primary care providers the flexibility to encounter participants in multiple settings as often as necessary to adequately manage their health problems.

In addition to managing participants from a biopsychosocial perspective, the PACE PCP must remain mindful of resource utilization. Federal rules and regulations require PACE organizations function as both the medical provider and insurance manager of the participant's health care benefits. This more directly aligns service provision with the cost of care and heightens the importance of quality care. Emphasizing prevention is a key task of the PACE PCP. In addition, an awareness of the cost/benefit associated with specific health services, medications, and DME is essential.

Care Coordination

As mentioned at the beginning of this chapter, care coordination across the continuum of care is vital to good outcomes for older adults. It is also a dying art form for medical providers. Increasingly, there are providers who specialize in particular sites/levels of care. This does ease the burden of practice management for many providers by delegating care to others at key times. However, delegation comes at significant price for patient care coordination, communication, and contributes to fragmentation of care. PACE medical providers realize the importance of involvement and communication with other providers. It does not mean that PACE providers serve as hospital and nursing home provider for every PACE participant. However, it does mean that providers prioritize involvement to the degree of essentially "co-management" of hospitalized PACE participants between hospital-based specialists and PACE medical providers. Staying updated on the evolution of medical status while hospitalized in key to a smooth discharge and transition to outpatient management. PACE medical providers are expected, by the very structure of PACE, to maintain an information pipeline between inpatient and outpatient providers.

End-of-Life Care

The eligibility criteria for PACE limits enrollment to a fairly complex and frail population of older adults. Most participants remain in the PACE program until death. That means that medical management will almost always include planning and providing care at the end of life. PACE programs rarely transition care into the traditional, Medicare Hospice benefit at end-of-life. They almost always remain in PACE (see Chap. 23). Therefore, medical providers in PACE become quite skilled at coordinating end-of-life care and offering advice to participants and families.

Care Planning

Although medical providers in other care settings tend to distance themselves from the official care planning process, PACE medical providers are "front and center" when it comes to care plans. There are several reasons for this more robust involvement. First, the Federal Regulations require that a medical provider participate in the interdisciplinary care process. This includes initial (enrollment) assessments, semi-annual assessments and all other decisions that require "team participation." Second, it is essential for achieving the goals of keeping participants at home. The medical provider's perspective and priorities for care must synchronize with the members of the team and be consistent with the participant's goals of care. This is best achieved through the IDT care planning process. Another important consideration is control of service utilization. Anticipation of potential medical issues in advance is a critical part of the care planning process which helps to control utilization (hospital and nursing home level care). Thus, PACE medical providers have multiple reasons to fully engage with care planning (see Chap. 21).

Billing/Coding

Most medical providers are familiar with the importance of billing and coding. In the US health care system, most providers are paid according to the type and frequency of direct encounters. In PACE, it is not the case. The capitated format eliminates that payment-per-encounter structure. However, PACE clinicians must be proficient at proper documentation of the evaluation and management of all medical conditions that impact risk adjustment. All encounters should include the most accurate, specific ICD diagnosis. This is particularly true at the time of semi-annual reevaluation. This offers the medical provider a consistent opportunity to thoroughly review all medical problems and that they are coded at the highest appropriate level.

Summary

Medical providers in PACE are essential members of the interdisciplinary team (IDT). They provide primary medical care and valuable input to the care coordination and utilization management of PACE participants. Physicians (MD or DO), nurse practitioners, and physician assistants can all serve the role of primary care provider according to Federal PACE regulations and this offers more flexibility to staffing and management of the IDT. Special training in geriatric medicine is valuable but not required for PACE clinicians to provide excellent primary care to this population of frail, medically complex older adults.

Suggested Reading

1. Center for Medicare and Medicaid Services, Department of Health and Human Services. Medicare and medicaid programs: programs of all-inclusive care for the elderly. 42 CFR Parts 423 and 460. 2021.
2. Segelman M, Szydlowski J, Kinosian B, et al. Hospitalizations in the program of all-inclusive care for the elderly. J Am Geriatr Soc. 2014;62:320–4.
3. Sairenji T, et al. Shifting patterns of physician home visits. J Prim Care Community Health. 2016;7:71–5.
4. Wieland D, Lamb VL, Sutton SR, et al. Hospitalization in the program of all-inclusive care for the elderly (PACE): Rates, concomitants, and predictors. J Am Geriatr Soc. 2000;48:1373–80.

Chapter 18
The Role of Medical Director in PACE

Catherine Eng

Introduction

The medical director is an essential leadership role in all health care practices and programs. Sometimes called "chief medical officer" (CMO) or lead physician, the skills and qualities are the same. These include an excellent fund of medical knowledge, excellent interpersonal skills, the ability to gain consensus from diverse disciplines, courage, and the ability to constructively deal with conflict. Additional skills that are helpful are an understanding and appreciation of finances and business aspects of the relevant program.

Overview of PACE Medical Director Role

As the lead medical administrator, the MedDir works closely with other senior leaders and usually reports directly to the CEO. Knowledge of organizational and Board structure is crucial to the success of the MD.

The MedDir must be knowledgeable of the PACE regulations and be prepared for CMS audits. In addition to the federal PACE regulations, the MD must also be knowledgeable of the State PACE regulations and local/county ordinances particularly in the area of Infection Control.

When a PO is small or at the start-up phase, the MedDir may be under contract for specified hours per week as a medical consultant to organize medical services.

C. Eng (✉)
On Lok Senior Health Services, San Francisco, CA, USA

Department of Medicine and Geriatrics, UCSF School of Medicine, San Francisco, CA, USA
e-mail: cathy@onlok.org; Catherine.Eng@ucsf.edu

M. K. McNabney (ed.), *Community-Based Integrated Care for Older Adults*,
https://doi.org/10.1007/978-3-031-05137-1_18

As the PO grows in enrollment and more primary care providers are recruited, the MedDir may become a full-time role.

The primary administrative responsibilities of the MedDir are organization of the medical staff, oversight of medical staff activities, oversight of the Quality improvement program, and utilization management.

Organization of the Medical Staff

Primary care providers including physicians and advance practice clinicians (APCs)—nurse practitioners and physicians assistants—must be hired. A staffing ratio of one PCP provider per 80–100 is a reasonable target for physicians and 50–60 enrollees per NP. A PO with fewer than 100 enrollees would typically hire a full-time physician PCP. When census reaches 150 enrollees, an NP could be hired instead of a half time physician. The functioning of APCs may vary by state regulations. For example, in some states, nurse practitioners are licensed independent providers; in other states, NPs are required to practice with, or under the guidance of a collaborating physician. PACE enrollees have complex chronic conditions, so a geriatrics-trained NP would be the best fit. The MedDir must set performance standards for the PCPs and APCs with measurable goals. In many states the APCs must adhere to a practice manual in addition to direct oversight by a physician.

In addition to the onsite primary care providers, the MedDir must recruit medical and surgical specialists under contract to serve as consultants to the PCPs. The consultant network must have every specialty represented, and the specialists must have privileges at the POs' contracted hospitals. Reimbursement for specialists is usually Medicare allowable and no co-pays to PACE patients must be explicitly indicated in the contract. Another feature of the contract should include services and procedures only as authorized by the PACE PCP and there can be no referrals by the specialist to other specialists without PACE PCP authorization. The MedDir must authorize any out of network provider services requested by the PCP. Further, the medical director interfaces closely with contracted subspecialists, and at times, must negotiate care that fits within the PACE model [which may be substantially different from local practice]. An essential role is to educate subspecialists in the ability of the PACE site to provide comprehensive, wrap around services, that assure quality of care even in locations of care that are not part of the traditional model of care delivery. Other than physician medical specialists, specialists such as dentists, optometrists, podiatrists, and audiologists can also be recruited, usually under contract, as these services are specifically required under PACE regulations. These specialty services can be provided on-site or in the specialist offices.

In addition, the MedDir participates in contract negotiations with local hospitals and skilled nursing facilities. In most states, hospital reimbursement rates for POs are usually Medicare DRGs. In some states, per diem rates are set and paid according to length of stay. Payments to skilled nursing facilities (SNF) are usually a Medicaid per diem rate. Other ancillary contracts include laboratory and durable medical equipment (DME) providers as well as home health agencies. All these providers must undergo proper credentialing, which falls under the Quality Improvement program as described below.

The scope of network development is quite extensive, and could well require a full time MedDir who does the network development half time while providing primary care half time until census is high enough to recruit a full time PCP.

Oversight of Medical Practice

The MedDir establishes practice guidelines and monitors medical staff adherence to those guidelines. The MedDir provides direct oversight of PCP practice and is responsible for annual written performance reviews. Practice guidelines typically include chronic conditions prevalent in frail older adults. These conditions include dementia, depression, heart failure, COPD, diabetes, renal failure, osteoporosis, atrial fibrillation and cerebrovascular disease. An additional practice guideline is preventive care, and includes immunizations such as pneumococcal, tetanus, influenza, and vaccination for herpes zoster as well as an advance directive for healthcare. Advance directives for healthcare should be obtained upon enrollment and reviewed annually. The semiannual reassessment is the perfect opportunity for the MedDir to review practice patterns among providers and to offer guidance towards practice improvement.

Clinical Coverage

Clinical coverage for all PACE enrollees must be carefully established (On-Call coverage) and disseminated to all providers of care who could need to reach the medical providers during nights and weekends. In-house PACE providers typically provide this coverage, but there could also be opportunity to integrate outside (non-PACE) providers into the call schedule to lessen the call burden by PACE providers. Of course, this requires that all cross-covering staff have a reasonable amount PACE knowledge and access to PACE providers as a form of back up. There must also be "quality control" regarding all medical providers participating in the clinical coverage scheme. This includes feedback from participants and families, as well as provider staff at any entity where the PACE program might have participants receiving care.

Medical Records

In the past several years, all PACE programs have transitioned to electronic health records (EHR). This was no easy process! However, there has been considerable progress and acclimation to the EHR as it pertains to the PACE model of care and regulatory requirements for documentation. The National PACE Association (NPA) has provided a great deal of support and collective guidance in this area. Major issues have included whether to maintain a completely separate EHR (for only PACE use) or to manage a PACE population within an EHR serving a larger health system. Needless to say, this is continuous work in-progress and each PACE program has distinct challenges that require the MedDir expertise and oversight with regard to medical records.

Quality Improvement Program

This is one of the most important responsibilities of the MedDir, after recruitment and retention of a primary care staff. The MedDir must lead in the creation of a comprehensive QI plan. The fundamentals of the plan are to gather practice data, measure adherence to practice guidelines, analyze results, and provide feedback for practice improvement. The MedDir hires QA analyst staff to assist in data analysis and report generation. The MedDir oversees the work of the QA staff and assures the findings are accurate. Most established POs have an electronic health record (EHR). There must be an IT staff and infrastructure to generate reports for data analysis. A robust QI program includes studies of common geriatric syndromes such as falls and management of pressure ulcers. An important aspect activity is medical care peer review which can be based on practice guidelines. Studies are done quarterly, and the results reported back to the medical staff.

An important aspect of the QI plan is Infection Control. The PO may need to hire an Infection Control nurse to manage the program with direct oversight by the MedDir. The Covid-19 pandemic has highlighted the importance of a robust infection program in long-term care to minimize spread of infection and mortality.

Provider credentialing is part of the QI plan. All providers, whether employed or under contract, must be properly credentialed, according to National Center for Quality Assurance (NCQA) guidelines. Elements of credentialing include maintenance of active licensure and certifications, possession of adequate levels of malpractice coverage. External databases are queried for each provider including National Practitioner Data Bank (NPDB) and Office of Inspector General (OIG). Credentialing might also include site visits to consultant offices or facilities to ensure adequate access for the disabled frail older adult.

Utilization Management

The MedDir monitors and manages utilization of costly services such as acute hospital admissions and 30 day readmissions (https://www.cms.gov/Research-Statistics-Data-and-Systems/Research/HealthCareFinancingReview/Downloads/CMS1191182dl.pdf). The financial viability of a PO depends on close oversite of hospital admissions and length of stay. The frail older adult population, in general, uses a disproportionate share of Medicare and Medicaid dollars primarily due to high hospital utilization. Efficient hospital utilization (and avoiding hospitalization when care could be provided in an alternative location of care) has been a hallmark of the PACE model since its inception. Upon enrollment in PACE, acute hospital care declines dramatically for this population due to efficient management by the medical staff and interdisciplinary team [1]. Compared to comparable dual eligible older adult populations, PACE continues to show reduced acute hospital admissions and reduced 30-day readmissions [2].

Most PO will pay hospitals using Medicare DRG rates per admission. Cost for each uncomplicated admission such as heart failure or pneumonia would have a DRG rate of $8–10K. More complex admissions cost upwards of over $50K. Thus, uncontrolled hospital utilization would consume the major share of a POs monthly capitation payments. The MedDir must monitor the frequency of one day hospital admission and be prepared to deny payment for one day stays that are not medically necessary. When utilization is high, the MedDir meets with the PCP staff to discuss strategies to lower utilization. Strategies employed could include use of Milliman Clinical guidelines (MCG) software that are evidence based and indicate whether an acute hospital admission meets guidelines for admission. The MedDir maintains close contact with the medical staff to achieve effective utilization of resources.

Another area of utilization monitoring is the use of medical and surgical specialists. PCPs who are not comfortable in management of chronic conditions will have a tendency to refer complex cases to specialists to manage. When high utilization of outside specialist occurs, it could mean that the PCP staff need further training and mentoring in complex case management.

Prescription drug utilization is another area to be monitored. The MedDir could hire a consulting pharmacist to review utilization and reduce polypharmacy. Medicare Part D is included in the PACE financing model. A formulary is not a requirement for PACE plans. The MedDir must evaluate the pros and cons of choosing to have a restrictive formulary and decide the optimal arrangement that PACE program. Management of pharmacy utilization is important to prevent polypharmacy and to control costs of specialty drugs. The medical director works closely with the medical staff and pharmacist, using principles of de-prescribing and avoidance of polypharmacy to both improve care and reduce adverse drug events in his frail elderly population.

Other Medical Director Functions

The importance of marketing and enrollment to a PACE program has been well-described elsewhere (see Chap. 6). It is quite important for the PACE MedDir to be actively involved in these efforts. Creating a positive presence in the community to instill confidence in the program is critical to program growth. Similarly, enrollment time can be stressful for the IDT as some team members are appropriately pushing enrollment and census growth, as other members are carefully scrutinizing care needs upon enrollment and the ability to manage a person safely in the community. The MedDir should display leadership in bringing these aspects together while pushing all efforts to expand enrollment.

The MedDir is often the face of the program to the community. She or he is expected to make presentations to community groups, medical groups, independent medical providers, the media, and policy makers. Thus, the MedDir must be an effective communicator and a persuasive presenter. These skills are not normally taught or developed during medical training, but most likely will be learned "on the job."

The MedDir also plays an important role in regulatory compliance and monitoring for Fraud, Waste, and Abuse. Along with the executive director, there should be standing meetings with recurring agenda items to assist the MedDir in fulfilling this role and to provide optimal protections to the program and its participants. All POs have mandatory grievances and appeals process. The MedDir plays a central role in directing the process and ensuring timely and thoughtful reviews. Similarly, it is the role of the MedDir to translate the findings into improved performance and quality of care provided to PACE participants.

Summary

The Medical Director position is critical to the success of the PACE organization. The responsibilities are numerous and substantial. They require a leader who is comfortable in leading as well as someone who is comfortable in working within a team, be it a team of medical providers, or a team of administrators. The recruitment of a skilled clinician leader is a top priority for a successful PACE Organization.

References

1. Sands LP, Wang Y, McCabe GP, et al. Rates of acute care admissions for frail older people living with met versus unmet activities of daily living. J Am Geriatr Soc. 2006;54:339–44.
2. Segelman M, Szydlowski J, Kinosian B, et al. Hospitalizations in the program of all-inclusive care for the elderly (PACE). J Am Geriatr Soc. 2014;62:320–4.

Chapter 19
The Role of Rehabilitation in PACE

S. Hanlon Newhall, June Nicholas, and Deny Stiassny

Introduction

With aging, multiple factors can impact one's quality of life: medical comorbidities, social and economic resources, environment and availability of support systems, access to medications, and food. The concept of *aging in place*—remaining in one's home as they age—carries worries and concerns, including activities of daily living, mobility, and overall safety. As discussed in other areas of this work, quality patient-centered care requires input from a variety of clinical team members.

As health challenges increase with age, state and local agencies can facilitate access to home health agencies and community resources. However, financial and eligibility barriers exist that may limit individual access to these services and increase the risk of hospitalization and/or institutionalization. Buhr et al. [1] studied the factors that led family members of people with dementia to choose placement in a nursing home. The most common reason chosen was "my loved one needed more advanced or skilled care than I could provide." In addition to limited mobility, difficult behaviors related to dementia also ranked highly as a reason for placement, specifically behavior dysregulation and psychotic symptoms. Van Rensbergen et al. [2] found diseases such as stroke, dementia, diabetes and mobility problems are only important risks for institutionalization if they cause functional disability, which leads to overwhelming caregiver burden and need for outside assistance.

In a traditional Medicare fee-for-service model of care, occupational and physical therapy services offer interventions in a variety of settings: home, outpatient care, acute inpatient and long-term care. Each of these settings work independently of one another, with separate teams of therapists. While Medicare is a nationwide benefit, eligibility requirements for Medicaid and private insurance

S. H. Newhall (✉) · J. Nicholas · D. Stiassny
Hopkins ElderPlus, Baltimore, MD, USA
e-mail: smyers33@jhmi.edu; jnichola@jhmi.edu

M. K. McNabney (ed.), *Community-Based Integrated Care for Older Adults*,
https://doi.org/10.1007/978-3-031-05137-1_19

does vary state by state. This results in significant barriers that can negatively impact an individual's success with safely remaining in the community. Barriers include lack of communication and continuity of care between care settings, financial limits to durable medical equipment, and access to ongoing rehabilitation treatment in the community or at home. As such, if a patient is hospitalized and requires post-acute care prior to or upon returning home, care providers in each setting may have limited opportunities for communication to adequately assess a patient's needs for continuity of care. As of this writing, Medicare has an annual monetary cap on outpatient physical therapy (PT), occupational therapy (OT) and speech and language pathology (SLP) services. To receive home care services, a patient is required to be homebound, at least temporarily. Adaptive equipment that may improve the success of remaining in the home setting may not be covered by insurances, such as ramps or bedside commodes, limiting the success of aging in place.

The limitations of the fee-for-service model are clearly evident in the one individual, EF, who is an example of how the PACE model can address these barriers to enable this individual to remain safely in the community. EF presented with a complex history of cerebral palsy (CP) and Polio as a child, and was cared for by an aging parent. Both knees had been surgically fused early in life and EF had been ambulatory up until recently. Once the parent passed away, EF moved in with a sister who continued to provide care. EF slept in an upstairs room of the sister's home, crawled up and down the interior stairs, but had been unable to leave the house due to the large number of brick exterior steps. Medicare paid for a custom wheelchair that was unable to be used outside the home due to the lack of a ramp. Environmental barriers created a burden to EF who was homebound, and to EF's sister who was unable to safely leave the patient unattended. Quality of life for both patient and caregiver was negatively impacted with an increased risk for institutional placement.

PACE Priorities: Rehabilitation and Aging in Place

The rehabilitation component of the PACE interdisciplinary team (IDT) consists of physical therapy (PT), occupational therapy (OT) and speech-language pathology (SLP), but for the purposes of this chapter, the primary focus will be on the role of OT and PT in community-based integrative care.

The Program of All-Inclusive Care for the Elderly (PACE) model receives capitated funding from Medicare and Medicaid, which covers all of its participants' healthcare needs. *This includes all rehabilitative services that are routinely covered by Medicare and Medicaid as well as those not traditionally covered but are felt to be necessary to achieve the participant's goals.* The PACE model avoids the fragmented care offered in a traditional (fee-for-service) health care setting that does not provide continuity between providers and post-hospital care, such as home care, skilled nursing facilities, and outpatient care. PACE therapists are able to follow their participants through close management and treatment in all of the above settings. In the PACE model, these services are integrated into the general care participants receive, which embraces a comprehensive approach to care.

The service model across PACE sites is similar although there is some variability in care management depending on whether the community is urban or rural. Additionally, the role of the occupational and physical therapist may differ among states depending on the governing body that regulates the state practice act regarding licensure for each discipline.

While the aging population is growing across the United States, the profile of a PACE participant differs from the average older adult. In order to be eligible for a PACE site, community dwelling older adults must be certified by the state as requiring nursing home level of care. In general, a PACE participant experiences more chronic conditions and is more likely to have dementia than non-PACE geriatric adults [3].

Beyond Fee-for-Service: Rehabilitation in PACE

The foundation of the PACE model is the belief that frail older adults with chronic care needs are best served in the community whenever possible. The model serves people who have complex, chronic conditions and dynamic needs that may require various services, which could include acute care to potentially long-term care placement. The overarching philosophy and ability to integrate care through the core members of the IDT (including occupational and physical therapists) allows for a more seamless transition along the continuum of care. This unique philosophy and practice provides a distinct opportunity to address barriers that are typically experienced in a fee-for-service care model.

In the PACE model, Rehabilitation services may be integrated into the daily milieu of PACE on an outpatient basis in the day health center (DHC). Therapy needs are determined by the individual care plan for each participant and adjusted as individual health changes occur (see Chap. 21). Treatment programs are adapted to these changes, and can be offered in contracted care settings (i.e. hospital, skilled nursing facility). Should clinical needs dictate a change of setting, PACE therapists serve as liaisons, monitoring therapies and offering recommendations as appropriate. Along with the IDT, PACE therapists may participate in discharge planning. If the plan is discharge home or to an assisted living facility (on a temporary or permanent basis), the therapists will provide direct care and education to the participant and caregiver during that transition.

The PACE model extends rehabilitation services into the home which provides a birds-eye view of challenges faced by participants and their caregivers in their home environment. OTs conduct *home safety evaluations* and provide information to the IDT about modifications and durable medical equipment needed to create a safer environment. PT can provide training in the home to the participant and caregiver for changes in mobility. Empirically speaking, home-based treatment can reduce the risk of falls and premature placement in an alternative setting.

If a participant is unable to attend the DHC due to a change in status or other environmental or mobility barriers, PACE services are delivered in the home setting (known as "PACE-at-home"). In this case, therapists will provide in-home care based on the need as outlined in the care plan. The care provided to the PACE-at-home population is distinct from the care provided by traditional home care therapists in that the participant treatments are provided from initial enrollment through end-of-life care.

As an all-inclusive model, PACE expands the conventional definition of assistive devices and durable medical equipment that would may not be supported in a fee-for-service model, to include all items that improve the quality of life, maximize independence and promote safety. This allows PACE therapists to provide items including grab bars, tub benches and use innovative equipment such as custom seating systems that can be modified to the participant's needs as postural and functional changes occur. In an urban area such as Baltimore, homes are typically row houses with both exterior and interior steps and therapists have promoted the use of stair climbers fastened to a wheelchair that help move the participant up and down stairs. In the case of EF, the team approved an electric stair climber to allow her to exit the home in her custom wheelchair. For someone who had been home bound for several years, this provided the opportunity for EF to reintegrate into the community, thus enriching her socialization and quality of life while also reducing caregiver burden.

Unlike the fee-for-service model, PACE supports placement of stair glides to navigate steps within the home setting when the team deems it is a necessary device to safely maintain the participant in the community and impact that individual's quality of life. Examples of other specialized equipment provided include a standing transfer aid, specialty walkers, lift chairs, specialty beds, and other unique durable medical equipment.

The Role of the Rehabilitation Department in PACE

Compared to the general geriatric adult population, geriatric adults served by PACE experience a greater complexity of medical and cognitive conditions. Rehabilitation professionals provide *assessments* for functional disability, as it relates to home accessibility, pain management, and fall and risk assessments. *Treatment interventions* follow in the form of mobility and strength training and treatment of various conditions including trauma recovery, and orthopedic, neurologic, and metabolic conditions. In situations of cognitive decline, OTs are able to help identify a participant's strengths that offer tools to guide caregivers in more effective ways to engage the person and thereby manage sometimes difficult behaviors and improve the quality of life for all.

PACE allows for PT/OT to be involved in the interdisciplinary team (IDT) decision-making process throughout the participant's enrollment Therapists are involved from pre-enrollment to end-of-life care. Starting at pre-enrollment, therapists complete an initial evaluation to identify client factors such as cognition and mobility, access to equipment and support, and safety barriers that may exist in the community and then present this information during the initial care plan. As part of the IDT, barriers and anticipated needs for participants to remain living in the community are discussed. Once enrollment is complete, a home safety evaluation is completed with recommendations for level/type of support, equipment, and home modifications that are recommended by the PACE program to maximize safety in the home and community. Then, therapists facilitate the ordering, delivery, and training of recommended equipment. Additionally, a home improvement vendor associated with the PACE program or one chosen by the participant is contracted to make appropriate home modifications to maximize safety in the home and allow access to the community.

Rehabilitation staff complete ongoing re-evaluations every six months to identify changes in mobility level, caregiver support, equipment needs, or need for additional skilled intervention. Throughout enrollment, therapists work closely with other team members to maintain participants in their home environment as much as possible. Unfortunately, when participants are unable to stay in their home, therapists are integral in the transition between settings. Additionally, throughout enrollment, PT and OT provide recommendations and intermittent consulting while participants are in care settings outside of PACE. Recommendations are made based on therapists' clinical judgment in the best interest of the participant. Generally, these recommendations are presented to the team for final approval. The overarching goal of rehabilitation is to maximize independence and safety in the community as long as possible.

Throughout PACE enrollment, rehab services are provided to participants in the PACE center and/or their home environment. Therapy services can include conservative pain management, equipment recommendations and training, mobility and transfer training, activity tolerance training, home safety, orthotics, and prosthetics. Special programs offered by rehabilitation department at PACE facilities vary site to site based on population need. In general, PACE rehabilitation departments offer specialized programs to meet the needs of PACE participants, including but not limited to fitness training, preventive medicine, wound care, lymphedema and chronic disease management. These interventions can be performed in individual or group settings. Further details of some of these specific programs with examples are described below.

Role of Rehabilitation in Falls Prevention and Home Safety

According to the Centers of Disease Control (CDC), falls are the most common cause of both traumatic brain injury and fractures in older adults [4]. Each year, three million older people are treated in emergency departments for fall-related injuries. Risk factors range from lower extremity weakness, mobility and balance skill difficulty, cognitive impairment, vision impairment, medications and polypharmacy, depression and the risk increases when these factors are combined [5]. Occupational therapists play an integral role in identifying risks and offering interventions in the way of home safety evaluations, cognitive assessment, and prescribing and implementing structured exercise and mobility training programs. Physical therapists provide functional outcome measures for balance and gait, mobility aids and tailored treatment programs to address joint, strength and balance limitations that impair one's mobility within home and the community. As already discussed, PACE therapists can also recommend and provide durable medical equipment not traditionally covered by Medicare fee-for-service to facilitate activities of daily and safe mobility. Many shared goals include energy conservation, sequencing motor tasks and caregiver training to improve safety. Members of the rehab team typically participate in any existing falls committee at a PACE site.

Role of Rehabilitation in Pain Management

Decline in mobility is expected with aging, and older adults with chronic pain experience a greater rate of functional mobility decline than their pain-free peers [6]. Both musculoskeletal and non-musculoskeletal pain may contribute to fall risk. Pain may also interfere with movement related parameters, such as strength, joint stability, flexibility, and reactive balance. In more chronic and complex scenarios, centralization of pain further complicates mobility performance due to development of fear-avoidance behaviors. Pain medication, while often effective, carries side-effects and risks. Daoust et al. concluded that recent opioid use is associated with an increased risk of falls in older adults and an increased likelihood of death in those with fall-related injuries [7]. In support of offering non-pharmacologic tools, conservative pain management interventions may be provided in the form of manual therapy, modalities, exercise, and patient education in joint protection. Additional modalities can include: moist heat, whole body vibration, adaptive yoga, mindfulness, and education and problem solving on energy conservation principles. These interventions are offered to mitigate the negative impact that pain has on an individual's functioning, i.e., mood, self-restriction of activity, and overall independence. In the PACE model of care, the rehab team is well positioned to work in cooperation with the medical providers, pharmacy, social work, nursing and recreation in identifying multi-faceted approaches to pain management. By addressing pain through conservative, alternative and traditional pain management modalities, the rehabilitation department with the entire IDT fosters preservation of functional mobility and independence in the community.

Occupational Therapy and Dementia/Cognition

As part of the core IDT, OTs play a vital role in the assessment and treatment of dementia and other types of cognitive impairment at PACE sites. A large number of individuals enroll in a PACE program with pre-established diagnoses such as dementia or mild cognitive impairment, and many exhibit challenging behaviors that impact their daily care and result in increased caregiver burden. Other individuals experience cognitive changes throughout their PACE enrollment, which are identified by a healthcare provider, family member or caregiver, and/or the participant. Cognitive changes may appear subtle, such as getting confused about the day of the week, but small changes in memory, executive functioning, and attention can lead to significant safety concerns. For example, an individual may notice forgetting items on the stove while cooking, which could lead to burns or a fire. Another individual may report a habit of misplacing medication bottles, which could result in issues with non-adherence or other medical complications. These concerns may be noticed by a nurse on the homecare team, a social worker checking in with a concerned caregiver, or a PT/OT during a home visit. Because of the nature of the consistent care that participants receive in a PACE program by a variety of providers, there are many opportunities to identify changes that impact an individual's ability to function safely in their home and community environments.

To assess an individual's level of functional cognition and ability to participate in activities of daily living, OTs use several different assessment tools such as the: Allen Cognitive Level Battery, the Kohlman Evaluation of Living Skills (KELS), and the Cognitive Linguistic Quick Test (CLQT). The type of assessment used depends on the concerns that arise from a team member, family, or participant about changes in functioning, i.e., ability to safely engage in self-care activities without assistance, prepare meals, or operate a power mobility device. The Allen Battery is an assessment tool that evaluates a person's ability to perform basic skills, problem solve, make decisions, and learn new abilities. It is administered through a screening tool using a lacing activity followed by a craft-based task. Results of these two activities are categorized into six levels of cognitive capabilities. These levels infer an individual's capacity to successfully engage in daily occupations. The KELS is a tool that measures areas of concern for safety in the home and community, in the areas of self-care, safety and health, money management, transportation and telephone, and work and leisure. Results on this assessment indicate potential need for assistance with integrating or reintegrating into their community. The CLQT is a short assessment that evaluates an individual's strengths and weaknesses in five cognitive domains: attention, memory, executive functions, language, and visuospatial skills. It is generally used to measure cognitive changes over time and can be used to inform the need for further assessment in specific cognitive areas.

The OT communicates the assessment and interpretation to the team to determine next steps. Interventions for cognitive changes may include implementation of tailored activity programs, issuance/training on use of durable medical equipment, or education and training about compensatory supports to help manage target behaviors and individual challenges. Below is a list of examples of interventions that may be put into place to address certain behaviors of individuals with cognitive decline:

Behavior/challenge	Intervention
Wandering at night, attempting to leave the home unaccompanied	Non-restrictive wandering banner (STOP sign), door or bed alarm
Forgetting to take medications on time	Training on compensatory memory tools, such as setting a phone alarm or timer
Stair navigation	Modifying stairwell by adding brightly colored tape to handrails and steps for depth and contrast
Safety during meal preparation/cooking	Providing an adapted microwave, stove knob covers, or an electric water heater to avoid stove use and reduce chances of a fire
Agitation and restlessness	Therapy dolls, sensory-based manipulatives such as stuffed animals, pat mat, and activity aprons, providing music, sensory books

Tailored Activity Programs

A tailored activity program (TAP) is a research-based OT intervention shown to decrease challenging dementia behaviors and caregiver burden. Individuals with dementia may exhibit challenging behaviors, including resistance to care, physical aggression, and wandering or exit-seeking behaviors. These behaviors place a significant burden on caregivers as they attempt to assist family members in completing daily self-care tasks. Based on an interview using an activity inventory with the caregiver and/or person with dementia, OTs design activities tailored to an individual's abilities and interests, and then train caregivers in using these activities as part of their daily routine. Activities could be designed to mirror household tasks such as folding laundry or washing dishes, or could be related to leisure activities such as floral arranging or playing card games. OTs develop tailored activities that align with a person's cognitive abilities and preserved interests to help redirect behavioral symptoms through meaningful activity engagement. Caregivers are often trained to implement these interventions in the home setting, although PACE care providers, such as medical technicians and patient aides, can also be trained to implement tailored activities at PACE sites. Customizing activities based on a wide range of physical, sensorimotor, and cognitive abilities provide opportunities for individuals with dementia to engage with their environments in a more meaningful way. After regular implementation of tailored activities, many caregivers report reductions in challenging behaviors and improved overall well-being in individuals with dementia.

Summary

The PACE model of care is a proactive and comprehensive approach for its participants, focused on preservation of function, quality of life, and supporting community-based care delivery. The overarching goal of PACE is to help participants with a common goal—"stay in the home you love." The rehabilitation team plays a vital role in supporting the health and well-being for frail older adults served by PACE. Rehabilitation services are developed at each PACE site to best suit the demographics and needs of the community.

References

1. Buhr GT, Kuchibhatla M, Clipp EC. Caregivers' reasons for nursing home placement: clues for improving discussions with families prior to the transition. Gerontologist. 2006;46:52–61.
2. Van Rensbergen G, Nawrot T. Medical conditions of nursing home admissions. BMC Geriatr. 2010;10:46.
3. https://www.npaonline.org/sites/default/files/PDFs/PACE-Quick-Facts.pdf.
4. https://www.cdc.gov/homeandrecreationalsafety/falls/adultfalls.html.
5. Hartley G, Kirk-Sanchez N. Fall risk in community-dwelling elders. APTA clinical summary. 2013.
6. Coyle PC, Schrack JA, Hicks GE. Pain energy model of mobility limitation in the older adult. Pain Med. 2018;19:1559–69.
7. Daoust R, Paquet J, Moore L, et al. Recent opioid use and fall-related injury among older patients with trauma. CMAJ. 2018;190:E500–6.

Chapter 20
The Role of Dietician-Nutritionist in PACE

Dana Kennedy

Introduction

Just as our bodies continue to change and evolve as we grow older, so do our nutritional needs to maintain our physical and cognitive function. The role of the Registered Dietitian remains critical throughout the human lifecycle and is crucial in the care of the older adult. Older adults are often at high nutritional risk, or high risk of malnutrition. **According to the World Health Organization, malnutrition may include *undernutrition*, which includes wasting, stunting and underweight; *micronutrient-related malnutrition* which includes micronutrient deficiencies; and *overweight, obesity and diet-related non-communicable diseases* (such as heart disease, stroke, diabetes and some cancers).**

There are multiple reasons for this risk and why interventions from a Registered Dietitian-Nutritionist (RDN) would be warranted. For example, as people grow older, they generally slow down physiologically. They are less active and more sedentary which can then lead to a decrease in appetite and food intake. This decrease in food intake can then lead to the slowing down of digestive processes, constipation, and dehydration. An RDN works to create an individualized plan to incorporate more calorically dense, high-fiber meals, snacks, beverages, and daily movement. This plan would promote good nutrition, hydration, and bowel motility. On the other hand, sometimes if older adults are more sedentary and less active, they may still eat just as much (or more) as when they were in the work force and more active. Food choices may also be less nutrient dense (think: junk food) due to boredom, low income, or lack of access to nutritious foods (think: fruits, vegetables, whole grains, and lean protein). This increase in less-nutritious energy (food) intake combined with decreased movement can lead to unintentional weight gain,

D. Kennedy (✉)
Community LIFE, Pittsburgh, PA, USA

M. K. McNabney (ed.), *Community-Based Integrated Care for Older Adults*,
https://doi.org/10.1007/978-3-031-05137-1_20

overweight/obesity leading to arthritis, acid reflux disease and depression. An RDN would work with this patient on an individualized plan to increase movement, substitute nutritious ingredients and foods with those of lesser nutrient value and hold the patient accountable for making sustainable, life-long behavior change versus following a short-term "fad" diet.

The Role of the Dietitian-Nutritionist in PACE

Working for a PACE program is extraordinarily rewarding because it allows staff to focus on what matters most to older adults—preservation of dignity, quality of life and promoting independence. But how does nutrition and the role of the registered dietitian-nutritionist (RDN) integrate into this model? To quote an anonymous speaker: "Nutrition is not low fat. It's not low calorie. It's not being hungry and feeling deprived. It's nourishing your body with real, whole foods so that you are consistently satisfied and energized to live life to the fullest." Like gasoline is to a vehicle, food is the fuel that gives our bodies the ability to function and perform activities of daily living. Quite literally, food = life. But food is more than that, is it not? **For many, food translates to love, care, memories, togetherness, warmth, comfort, fun, family, friends and celebrations**. Food and nutrition are just as uniquely personal as they are universal, and they are vital components to living a full, happy and healthy life—the same approach to life that we strive to promote for participants.

As the Registered Dietitian-Nutritionist in a PACE program, **it is critical to understand how food affects participants from a medical, social and financial standpoint**. Balancing that fine line between recommending nourishment that people want and what people need is equally important. At the end of the day, after the pills are swallowed, personal care is completed and durable medical equipment is parked, what other choices are left up to participants? **Recognizing that the mission of PACE is to enable frail, older adults to remain at home while preserving their dignity, independence and quality of life, the mission of the RDN is to assess how food and nutrition can help participants to achieve their specific goals so they can remain living in the community**. Whether these goals are geared toward longevity, maintaining current function, or comfort care, the RDN integrates with the interdisciplinary team to care plan and monitor the effectiveness of nutrition interventions. The role of the RDN in PACE is expansive and quite different from other models of care; thinking outside-the-box is preferable and it all starts with meeting the participants where they are on their journey.

From an interdisciplinary team (IDT) standpoint per the PACE regulations, the Registered Dietitian-Nutritionist represents one of the eight mandatory disciplines who must complete a comprehensive in-person nutrition assessment upon initial enrollment, semiannually (if represented on the care plan), annually, if a re-assessment is ever requested by the participant and/or family and upon significant change in health or psychosocial status. As a mandatory IDT member, based on information provided from the nutrition assessment and the participant's specific goals, the RDN may formulate a nutritional problem, goal(s) and intervention(s) for the participant to work toward over the next six months. Let us go back to the participant who has a decreased appetite and calorie intake due to physiologic decline, and let us call this participant Mr. Jones. A specific nutritional problem for the care plan may be that Mr. Jones is at risk for unintentional weight loss and dehydration due to decreased appetite and intake of meals, snacks and beverages. A SMART (specific, measurable, attainable, realistic and time-sensitive) goal for Mr. Jones could be that he will have no unintentional significant weight loss (greater than or equal to 10% of current body weight) over the next six months. Another goal could be that Mr. Jones will remain adequately hydrated as evidenced by lab work as ordered and no signs or symptoms of dehydration (example: dry mouth, excessive thirst, dark-colored urine). The interventions for the care plan are what reflects the true interdisciplinary nature of the PACE model. This is because while the RDN will be providing nutrition education/counseling and likely nutritional supplements to the participant for home use, other disciplines will be playing a role in keeping Mr. Jones stable as well. The nurse will weigh the participant on a monthly basis, the provider will order lab work, evaluate medications and assess in the clinic as needed, the day center will provide meals, snacks and beverages on his specific days of attendance, the home-care supervisor will oversee the home health aides who provide meal prep in the home as needed, and the physical therapist will encourage increased movement to support appetite stimulation.

In-Person Nutrition Assessment

Food is a funny thing. It can spark memories and stories that lead into hour-long conversations about why on Earth someone cannot stand to look at a piece of asparagus or a bowl of oatmeal. It can also initiate beautiful moments of reminiscing between the RDN and a participant with Alzheimer's Dementia—someone who cannot remember what he ate for breakfast that morning but can remember, in the finest of details, what it was like to work on his grandfather's farm when he was 10 years old. Comprehensive, face-to-face nutrition assessment may occur in the PACE center, skilled nursing facility or in the participant's home. Routine assessments are done at enrollment, annually, semiannually and when there is a significant change in the participant's health, medical or psychosocial status. This is when the RDN collects invaluable data. This data includes the participant's ability to cook and/or plan and prepare simple meals with functioning kitchen facilities. We assess the participant's ability to independently grocery shop—many need assistance with either transportation, finances or home-delivered meals. **The RDN assesses a participant's dietary habits, meal pattern, average oral intake, and nutritional supplement use** (if indicated). Assessments include not just what participants eat but also *how* they eat with current dentition—if they have difficulty chewing or swallowing or other digestive issues. "How" a participant eats may also refer to the ability to feed themselves independently, if they need adaptive dining equipment or if they require assistance from a family member or caregiver to eat. Food preferences, including likes, dislikes and religious/ethnic restrictions are noted as well as any specific food allergies, intolerances, sensitivities or diversions. Recognizing that other lifestyle factors play a role in an individual's nutritional status, the RDN assesses if the participant smokes tobacco, uses other illicit drugs, drinks alcohol and/or engages in regular physical activity throughout the day. The RDN must evaluate several factors which may indicate whether a participant has increased or decreased caloric, macronutrient/micronutrient or fluid needs. This includes vital clinical data such as diagnoses, medications, lab values, skin status (pressure injuries) and weight. It is with a full, comprehensive face-to-face nutrition assessment that the RDN can collaborate with the participant and IDT to make the most appropriate recommendations for the care plan.

Nutrition Requirements & Interventions for the PACE Population

After training and board certification, Registered Dietitians are prepared to direct people on eating healthy foods, practicing portion control, movement, maintaining a healthy weight and changing their lives for the better. Confident in the ability to stay positive and help people achieve their health and wellness goals, RDNs face a deep reality check in the real world. With experience, RDNs come to realize that there is a tremendous gap between what people *think* it means to eat healthy and balanced and what it *actually* means to eat healthy and balanced. During encounters with participants, RDNs have to typically tread lightly, earn trust and most importantly listen as participants describe a typical day of meals, snacks, desserts and beverages. Some participants describe diets that they have considered, or followed, which are overly restricted or otherwise unhealthy for that person. Some people hear the word "diet" and automatically think "deprivation" or "starvation" or having to give up favorite foods forever. **PACE participants are living in the community with the freedom and ability to make their own choices and that includes food and drink**. The RDN in a PACE setting is responsible for educating participants about their individualized nutritional needs and providing the means to help them meet those requirements safely. Monthly weight monitoring is one measurement tool RDNs use to assess whether or not a participant is meeting his or her nutritional requirements. While weights may fluctuate due to other factors including edema/fluid retention, weight change may also reflect nutritional problems including inadequate protein-calorie intake or muscle wasting. It is important that the RDN monitor for significant weight change for quality auditing purposes as well. "Significant" weight change is defined as 5% gain or loss in 30 days, 7.5% gain or loss in 90 days and 10% gain or loss in 180 days. Upon identifying those participants who have had an unintentional significant weight change, the RDN as well as other disciplines can either do a re-assessment (if indicated) and/or revise the care plan to include appropriate goals and interventions. One way in which the PACE model provides these nutrition interventions is by serving two meals and one to two snacks daily in the adult day centers to those who are attending. As supervisors of the dining service assistants, the RDN oversees the purchasing of meals that are either prepared in-house or purchased from an outside foodservice vendor for holding and serving. Meal requirements for PACE participants can be found under the CMS (Centers for Medicare and Medicaid) PACE guidelines, as well as state-specific requirements of Departments of Aging (ex: Aging Program Directive for Congregate Meals). As an example from the Participant Nutrition Policy at the PACE site in Pittsburgh, PA: "Community LIFE provides food that is nourishing, palatable, well-balanced and meets acceptable safety standards. Menus are reviewed by Registered Dietitians to ensure recommended population standards are upheld." Standards for meals include requirements for amounts and types of protein, fruits and vegetables, grains or enriched bread, milk or other source of calcium, fiber, fat, sodium, vitamin C, vitamin A, calorie/energy level, potassium and optional dessert. Providing these meals in the day center provides the perfect gateway to educating participants on what it means to eat an overall healthy, balanced diet. The RDN is then able to help the participant build the connection between what they eat, how they feel and how nutrition plays a role with their overall medical diagnoses and care.

The structure and mission of PACE allows the RDN to get to know each participant individually and think outside of the box to explore the most appropriate interventions for his or her own journey. Unlike skilled nursing facilities or hospitals, therapeutic diets—diets that are prescribed to treat a variety of chronic illnesses including diabetes, chronic kidney disease, and cardiovascular disease—are not typically used or recommended in the PACE setting. To quote the Pioneer Network's New Dining Practice Standards and the position of the Academy of Nutrition and Dietetics on therapeutic diets, "the quality of life and nutritional status of older adults…can be enhanced by individualization to less-restrictive diets. Although therapeutic diets are designed to improve health, they can negatively affect the variety and flavor of the food offered. Individuals may find restrictive diets unpalatable, resulting in reducing the pleasure of eating, decreased food intake, unintended weight loss and undernutrition—the very maladies health care practitioners are trying to prevent. In contrast, more liberal diets are associated with increased food and beverage intake. For many older adults…the benefits of less-restrictive diets outweigh the risks." Does this mean that providing medical nutrition therapy, one of the foundational responsibilities of being a clinical dietitian is unimportant in a PACE setting? Does this mean that all participants should be free to eat whatever they want and be told that? That depends. In my experience, if you give people the education, the freedom of choice, a listening ear and autonomy, they will be much more likely and willing to work with you as the nutrition professional and not run from you as the food police.

Creative and Hands-on Approaches to Nutrition Education & Intervention

There are three things that participants seem to particularly appreciate from their interdisciplinary team (IDT)—our attention, our focus on keeping them independent in the community and the education that we provide so that they or their families can care for them. From a nutritional standpoint, **it is important (and mandatory) that we ask questions, complete assessments, provide meals and attend care conferences**. But **there are other more creative, fun and outcomes-based strategies to provide attention and user-friendly information to participants, such as providing small nutrition support groups and cooking demonstrations to participants**. Participants who have a vested interest in being more mindful about their diets and food choices can enjoy an hour's worth of group discussion on various topics including how to say no to "food pushers," how to determine hunger vs. cravings, how to prevent dehydration, how to read food labels and how to eat to help boost brain activity and memory. Nutrition support groups have also featured different recipes and sample tastings including smoothie recipes and a "build-your-own-power-bowl" with an assortment of healthy grains, proteins and vegetable sources. Cooking demonstrations which are typically executed separately include recipes that require little-to-no cooking equipment/kitchen facilities, few simple ingredients commonly found in pantries and inexpensive ingredients which can easily be obtained from food banks or local grocery stores. These recipes take minimal cooking (if required at all) and preparation time. It can be quite fun to put on the "Food Network Host" hat, get up in front of participants and put nutrition on the spotlight for an hour every month. The hands-on demonstration of how to prepare simple, palatable recipes is much appreciated by all of the participants because they can experience exactly what they are being taught in-person and in a multi-sensory way—seeing the chopping and mixing necessary for preparation, smelling the aromas of the different ingredients, touching a specific food or ingredient that they may have never bothered picking up previously at the store before and of course, the best part—tasting the final product! Every participant walks away with a recipe, the nutrition facts per serving of that recipe and the health benefits of incorporating the recipe into their meal and snack patterns.

Summary

The RDN plays an important role in the PACE model. As a required member of the IDT, the RDN must conduct regular nutritional assessments on each participant and make recommendations that are consistent with the goals of care and can be incorporated into the individual's care plan to help achieve goals that are person-specific and promote quality of life.

Suggested Reading

Pioneer Network Food and Dining Clinical Standards Task Force: New Dining Practice Standards. https://www.pioneernetwork.net/wp-content/uploads/2016/10/The-New-Dining-Practice-Standards.pdf

World Health Organization: Malnutrition. http://www.who.int/news-room/fact-sheets/detail/malnutrition

Part V
Special Aspects of the PACE Model

Chapter 21
Care Planning in PACE

Lisa Jenkins

Introduction

"Plan your work and work your plan." Whether talking about schoolwork, our careers, upcoming vacations, yard work or care for our participants, pausing to lay out a solid plan before diving into a project is key to success. "Failing to plan is planning to fail," as the adage goes.

A solid care plan lays a strong foundation for successful individualized care of PACE participants. Care planning is the process of assessing an individual, setting goals and determining how those goals will be achieved. It results in a written document—the care plan—that directs service delivery [1]. Used widely throughout medical and social services, care plans are critical is assisting both clients and their providers to set and achieve individualized goals built on the client's strengths and available resources. Care plans are a partnership between the individual and the provider empowering the individual to be a part of the care.

The concept of care planning was first formalized within the medical field in 1930 by Ellen L. Buell, a Public Health Nurse and Founder of the Department of Public Health Nursing in the College of Medicine at Syracuse University. Buell wrote in an article published in The American Journal of Nursing, "Thus it is that the steps in the process of solving any problem are stressed in the analysis of a family health problem; namely **the recognition of the problem, definite outlining and defining of the problem, formulation of possible solutions of the problem, selecting the solution which in this particular situation seems most feasible, application of the solution chosen, and finally judging the results in terms of its failure or its success**." [2]. As the care planning process was studied and refined

L. Jenkins (✉)
Supportive Care Services, Community LIFE, Pittsburgh, PA, USA
e-mail: jenkinslh@upmc.edu

M. K. McNabney (ed.), *Community-Based Integrated Care for Older Adults*,
https://doi.org/10.1007/978-3-031-05137-1_21

over the following years, Buell identified the important role that the patient has in partnering with the medical professional to implement the care plan. She wrote in a 1941 article that it is the responsibility of professionals "to formulate an acceptable plan for the protection and promotion of (the patient's) own health, and to encourage (the patient) to carry out the plan." [3].

Care planning was introduced to the world of long-term care in the late 1980s. The Omnibus Reconciliation Act of 1987, also known as the Federal Nursing Home Reform Act, instituted a wide range of changes to improve the quality of care in nursing homes and the quality of life for their residents. These changes included the formalization of assessing residents and using those assessments to develop individualized care plans [4].

PACE, founded in the early 1970s on the need for long-term care services outside of a nursing home for eligible older adults enables programs to "provide the entire continuum of care and services to seniors with chronic care needs while maintaining their independence in their home for as long as possible." [5]. **An individualized plan of care for each Participant guides the care and services provided.**

Care Plans in the PACE Model

Every PACE participant has a care plan—a written document laying out how the interdisciplinary team's (IDT) plans to provide and coordinate care. **Care plans are "living, breathing documents" meaning that they change, adapt, and grow as a participant's need change over time**. The CMS (Federal) PACE Regulations Subpart 460.106 [6] outlines instructions of when and how care plans are to be completed. Throughout this chapter, references to the specific sections of regulations are noted in parentheses.

When Is a Care Plan Completed?

According to the regulations, a Participant's initial care plan must be written "**within 30 days of the date of enrollment**" (Subpart 460.106a). After the initial care plan, "**on at least a semi-annual basis, the interdisciplinary team must reevaluate the plan of care, including defined outcomes, and make changes as necessary**" (Subpart 460.106d). Assessments for these care plans must be completed by the entire IDT.

A key word in this regulation is "at least." The regulations state that a comprehensive assessment of the participant needs to take place "on at least a semi-annual basis or more often if a participant's condition dictates" (Subpart 460.104c).

Updating the care plan based on change is one of the most powerful aspects of the PACE model. If a participant has a change of status (for example moves to a new apartment or has a significant medical decline), regulations direct that the IDT does not wait for the next scheduled review period to review and update the care plan. When a change of status occurs, in-person assessments are to be completed minimally by the primary care provider, a registered nurse, and master's level social worker as well as any other IDT member the team feels necessary (460-106c). The care plan is then reviewed and revised by the entire IDT, adapting services to fit the new needs of the participant. Each individual PACE program will have set criteria for the timeframe for a care plan driven by a change of status and for determining the specific staff to be involved in conducting assessments. The important thing to remember is that care plans are looked at in real time. Adjustments are made and needed services are provided when they are needed—not 2 weeks later.

The two scenarios listed above involve assessments being completed by the entire IDT. There is also a time when a care plan revision can be completed by a single discipline and reviewed by the entire IDT versus the entire IDT needing to do an assessment. For example, if a participant is seen in the clinic for a wound that is assessed to require significant care by the primary care provider and nurse, the nurse will write a care plan revision. The nurse will bring that care plan to the IDT for review. Other members of the IDT may have suggestions for care to add to the revision. In this case, the dietician may recommend a supplement to aid in the healing of the wound. Once the IDT has approved the revision, the author of the revision reviews it with the participant and/or caregiver (460-106e).

How Is a Care Plan Created?

The CMS (Federal) PACE regulations also provide directions on to how to write a care plan. Specifically, care planning can be broken down into six steps (see Table 21.1).

It is important to note that the involvement of the participant and/or primary caregiver is critical in the development of the care plan. In fact, it is so important that PACE programs are responsible for demonstrating and documenting how the participant and/or primary caregiver have been involved as specified in Subpart 460.106E of the federal regulations: "*Participant and caregiver involvement in plan of care.* The team must develop, review, and reevaluate the plan of care in collaboration with the participant or caregiver, or both, to ensure that there is agreement with the plan of care and that the participant's concerns are addressed." Demonstration

Table 21.1 Six steps to writing a care plan

1	Identify the needs/problems of the participant
2	Set measurable goals to address each problem
3	Determine how the goals will be met
4	Determine who will be responsible for each step
5	Set a date by which the goal must be met
6	Review the plan with the participant

and documentation of how that directive is carried out may be differ with each PACE program.

The following patient story will be used as we explore each of the six steps listed above:

Beverly is an 85-year-old widowed female who lives alone in her own home. She is alert and oriented times three. Beverly has a strong motivation to remain at home. She is proud of her home and holds tight the memories within her home. To accommodate her physical needs, her dining room has been transformed into a bedroom so that she does not need to climb the steps. There is a bathroom on the first floor, but no shower. Beverly has a long list of medical diagnosis which includes osteoarthritis, spinal stenosis, cervical disc disorder, hypertension, atrial fibrillation, GERD, anxiety disorder, major depressive disorder and obesity. She has a history of falls. Beverly has a cousin who is her sole support other than her PACE Team. She attends the Day Center 5 days a week. She receives homecare services twice a day 7 days a week to assist with personal care, housekeeping and meal preparation due to her physical limitations and chronic pain. Beverly manages her own finances with the oversight of her cousin; however, she has maxed out several credit cards through catalog shopping. Besides memory-filled antiques, her home is filled with unopened packages of clothes, jewelry and other as-seen-on-TV gadgets such that the walkways within the home are beginning to be compromised. The IDT has identified multiple factors which increase her anxiety such as changes in her homecare schedule, not having enough incontinence supplies, any mail from companies not familiar to her and falls. The IDT has noted that when her anxiety is increased, her falls also increase.

Step One: Identify the Needs/Problems of the Participant

Identifying the needs/problems/strengths of the participant is achieved after all the members of the IDT have completed an in-person discipline-specific assessment with the participant. Information may also be gathered from additional sources such as family members, contracted professionals and other PACE staff outside of the IDT. Team members take turns sharing the results of their assessments in a structured interdisciplinary care plan (ICP) that includes open discussion regarding the team's findings. **The IDT then works to reach a consensus of what problem(s) the care plan will focus on** (Subpart 460, 106.b1). Considering the complex population of older adults who are served by PACE, the potential problem list in the care plan can be very long. The team needs to decide which problems, diagnosis or concerns are the priority for that participant at this current time. Sometimes the list of problems comes together very quickly; at other times, there is great discussion and debate around the table. The IDT care planning discussion varies per participant, which is part of the beauty of the PACE model. There is personalized attention to each care plan by a team of dedicated and passionate health care providers. It should not simply be a "formality."

Looking at Beverly's scenario, what problems might be identified? Her team has combined several issues to identify one problem for her: History of falls complicated by pain, arthritis in multiple joints, and anxiety. You may ask yourself, what about her finances? If she is maxing out credit cards, is there not the potential problem of her not being able to pay her bills? A former Medical Director of one PACE program shared this insightful perspective: Who is it bothering? In this moment, her spending habits are not impacting her ability to live safely in the community. It is important to be aware of it, but that is not an active situation that is impacting her health. Who is her spending bothering? It appears to primarily bother members of the team. Beverly is not bothered by her spending habits at all; therefore, the IDT does not include concerns about her finances in the care plan.

Step Two: Set a Goal Addressing Each Problem

This is the key moment in establishing the participant's care. **The quality of the goal lays the groundwork for a solid care plan.** The goals direct the care being received and the services being provided. See Fig. 21.1 for more information on setting SMART goals.

While there is often considerable debate within the IDT about identifying the problems, the determination of the goal is a time of brainstorming with team members playing off one another throwing out phrases and ideas until the perfect goal is developed. As time goes on, a team may develop a list of "go to" goals that can be adapted to fit common scenarios and personalized to fit each individual participant. **It is important to consistently be referring to the question of "Is this a SMART goal?"** (Subpart 460.106.b2).

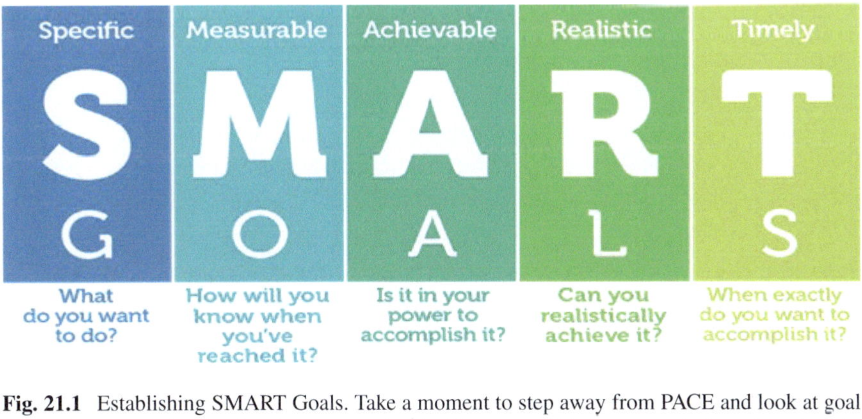

Fig. 21.1 Establishing SMART Goals. Take a moment to step away from PACE and look at goal setting in general. Goal setting is a core part of health care, so it is important to know how to set a solid *SMART* goal. (*Reprinted from V-Comply (May 31, 2019) SMART Goals are at the heart of every organization. https://blog.v-comply.com/smart-goals-for-business/)

Beverly's identified problem was: ***History of falls complicated by pain, arthritis in multiple joints, and anxiety****. The goal set to help her with that problem was:* ***Beverly will have no falls with serious injuries over the next 6 months.***

Specific? *Check—no falls with serious injuries.*

Measurable? *Check—This goal has a simple yes or no measurement. Beverly will suffer a serious injury or not.*

Achievable? *Check—the team feels that with their physical and emotional support and Beverly's motivation to remain in her home, that she has the power to accomplish this goal.*

Realistic? *Check—While the team is confident in the interventions they have put into place, they know that a PACE program is a risk-bearing program. They feel that there is a high probability that Beverly will fall; however, the hope is that the interventions will prevent a serious injury.*

Timely? *Check—This goal will be met within the next 6 months.*

Step Three: Determine How the Goal Will Be Met

Once the team has identified the problems and the goals they hope to achieve, it is **time for the IDT to talk about what needs to be done to help the participant achieve that goal.** What PACE services need to be started? What referrals need to be made? What interventions will the team put into place (Subpart 460–106.b3, 4, 5) for Beverly? See Table 21.2 for examples.

Step Four: Determine Who Will Be Responsible to Complete or Monitor Each Task

Once it is determined what needs to happen, **the IDT determines who is responsible for completing or monitoring each task.** See Table 21.3 for examples. There are several things to consider

- There could be more than one discipline assigned to a single task.
- Not all disciplines may be represented on each problem.
- One discipline could be assigned to multiple tasks under one problem.

Table 21.2 Problem/Goal/Interventions

Problem	Goal	What needs to happen
History of falls complicated by pain, arthritis in multiple joints, and anxiety.	Beverly will have no falls with serious injuries over the next 6 months	Provide homecare. Laundry services at day center Medications for pain Light housekeeping for fall prevention Provide durable medical equipment for fall prevention Wellness for strengthening and endurance Provide emotional support for anxiety

Table 21.3 Problem/Goal/Interventions/Responsible Parties

Problem	Goal	What needs to happen	Who is responsible
History of falls complicated by pain, arthritis in multiple joints, and anxiety	Beverly will have no falls with serious injuries over the next 6 months	Provide homecare for fall prevention	Home Care Coordinator
		Laundry services at day center for fall prevention	Home Care Coordinator
		Medications for pain	Primary Care Physician/RN Case Manager
		Light housekeeping for fall prevention	Home Care Coordinator
		Provide durable medical equipment for fall prevention	Occupational Therapist
		Wellness for strengthening and endurance	Occupational Therapist/ Physical Therapist
		Provide emotional support for anxiety	Master's Level Social Worker

From this example, it is often obvious which IDT members are expected to complete or monitor each task and document in the medical record. For example, looking at Beverly's care plan, the Home Care Coordinator is the appropriate person to monitor that homecare is being provided rather the Social Worker. Other times there may be more discussion about who should be assigned. Although every staff member who meets Beverly is going to be providing emotional support should she become anxious during their interaction, the team has determined that best discipline to be responsible for ensuring that the task is the social worker.

Step Five: Set a Date by Which the Goal Must Be Met

The determination of the date by which a goal should be met is often determined by the date of the next time the care plan will be reviewed. For PACE programs that date is determined by one of three things. First, CMS (Federal) PACE regulations and individual PACE program requirements. Federal regulations require PACE to re-assess the participant and revise the care plans every 6 months (460-106d). Second, individual PACE programs may require care plans to be reviewed and revised more often. Third, if a care plan revision is being made for a specific situation such as a respite stay in a nursing home or a wound, the goal's date will be determined by the details of that situation.

Step Six: Review the Care Plan with the Participant and/or the Primary Caregiver

As stated earlier, it is part of the Federal regulations that **the care plan is reviewed with the participant and their caregiver "to ensure that there is agreement with the plan of care and that the participant's concerns are addressed"** (460-106e). How this is accomplished and who is responsible will differ between PACE programs.

Six months later or when there is a change, this process starts again from Step One. It is a perpetual cycle of assess, review, revise and implement that continues for the duration of the time that a participant is a member of the PACE program. Earlier, care plans were referred to as living, breathing documents. This never-ending cycle illustrates how the care plans change, adapt, and grow as a participant's needs change over time. The infinite cycle also ensures that a high quality of care is being delivered as the Team is constantly assessing the progress of the participant and the Team in achieving the goals set in the care plan.

Documentation of the Care Plan in the PACE Model

CMS (Federal) PACE Regulations clearly state that **the care plan must be documented in the participant's medical record.** The actual care plan document itself must be in the medical record. There are several documentation formats that can be used which allow a program to meet the criteria laid out in the regulations. Each individual PACE program will need to determine which format is best. Specific disciplines are also required to document on interventions that they are responsible for within the care plan as they are putting those interventions into action. This continuous documentation of the care plan also demonstrates how a care plan is a living, breathing document. It is constantly being looked at and evaluated to ensure that the best care is being provided. Each PACE Program will determine exactly what that documentation will look like and how it is completed.

Summary

Back in 1930, Ellen Buell had a vision for creating a tool to assist nurses in connecting with their patients through completing assessments and setting individualized goals built on the patient's strengths and available resources. Today, PACE programs continue to carry on that partnership between the individual and the IDT empowering the individual to be an active part of the care while ensuring a high quality of care is delivered by the IDT.

References

1. McClam T, Woodside M. The helping process: assessment to termination; 2012. p. 111.
2. Buell E. The case study: as a method of teaching students and graduates the principles of public health nursing. Am J Nurs. 1930;30(4):399–407. https://doi.org/10.2307/3411154.
3. Buell E. Public health nursing—a contribution to the community health program. Pi Lambda Theta J. 1941;20(2):61–3.
4. Turnham H. OBRA '87 Summary. n.d.. https://www.ncmust.com/doclib/OBRA87summary.pdf

5. National PACE Association. The history of PACE. n.d.. https://www.naponlie.org/policy-advocacu/value-pace
6. CMS (Federal) PACE Regulations (Subparts 460–104 and 460–106). https://ecfr.io/Title-42/cfr460_main

Chapter 22
Care Coordination and Transitions of Care in PACE

Sarah Babineau

Transitions of care is defined as the movement of a person from one care setting to another when their health condition or care needs change. *Care coordination* is patient-centered, deliberate communication and coordination among members of a care team (including the person receiving care and their caregivers) to optimize and provide appropriate, safe, and effective care (see Fig. 22.1). Older adults are particularly vulnerable to errors when health information is not properly exchanged between settings. Studies have shown that poor transitions (as a consequence of inadequate care coordination) are associated with increased rates of potentially avoidable hospitalizations, re-hospitalization, and higher costs to the Medicare system.

There are several evidence-based transitions of care models which provide comprehensive care coordination across settings. The Care Transitions Program® under the leadership of Eric Coleman, MD, MPH, has developed several tools including the Care Transitions Intervention® (CTI). This intervention pairs patients with complex care needs and their caregivers with a Transitions Coach® who helps teach them skills to manage their health conditions. Dr. Mary Naylor and her team have developed and studied the Transitional Care Model. This program provides chronically ill older hospitalized adults with comprehensive discharge planning and home follow-up coordinated by a "Transitional Care Nurse". Both models have been shown to improve patient outcomes including reduced readmission to the hospital and decreased total healthcare costs as well as improved health and quality of life outcomes.

Poor communication and a lack of effective care coordination between settings are associated with medication errors, delays in follow up after hospitalization, and poor satisfaction with care. In a survey by the Commonwealth Fund,

S. Babineau (✉)
Providence ElderPlace, Seattle, WA, USA
e-mail: sarah.babineau@providence.org

M. K. McNabney (ed.), *Community-Based Integrated Care for Older Adults*,
https://doi.org/10.1007/978-3-031-05137-1_22

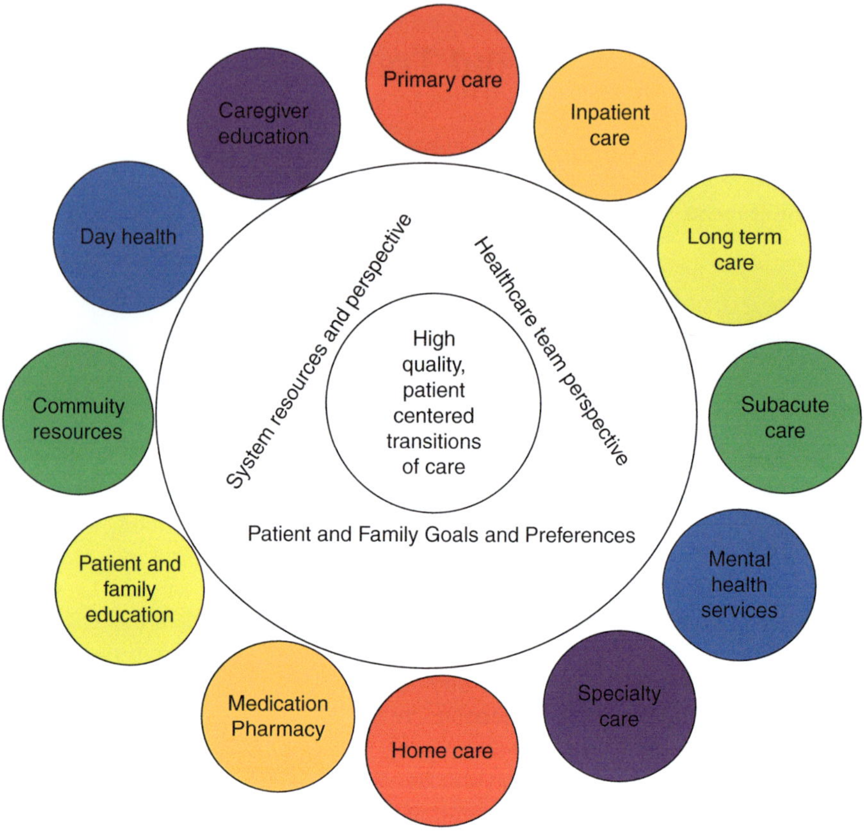

Fig. 22.1 Patient-Centered Transitions of Care. (Adapted from: https://itethertech.com/2019/08/30/what-is-care-coordination/)

half of "high-need" adults (defined as an individual 65 and older with at least 3 chronic conditions or a functional limitation in activities of daily living) experienced a problem with care coordination. This included test results either not being ready or duplicate tests being ordered, receiving conflicting information from doctors, and miscommunication between specialists and primary care providers.

Care models that are successful in minimizing the risks that occur during transitions of care have several components. These include **multidisciplinary care with coordination across settings, 24/7 availability of staff to respond to patient care needs, comprehensive patient assessment with evidence-based care planning which aligns with patient care goals, and prompt follow-up**. Close communication and proactive monitoring of health status across care settings are also necessary components of a successful transition. These components are all at the heart of the PACE model of care. In addition, PACE organizations are Medicare Part D providers and thus provide medications for their participants. Medication reconciliation is performed anytime a participant moves from one setting to another. PACE programs coordinate transportation to the PACE center and medical clinic as well as to specialty appointments. PACE providers work closely with specialists and follow up on specialty appointments and recommendations if appropriate for their participants' goals of care. The PACE model is designed to tailor services to the individual needs and goals of the patient.

Features of Successful Care Models

- Multidisciplinary teamwork
- Care coordination across settings
- Medication management and reconciliation
- Multi-dimensional assessment and care planning
- Alignment of care with patient goals
- Responsiveness 24/7 and prompt follow-up
- Education and engagement of patients and care partners
- Transitions of care seamless across settings

Adapted from: Long P, et al. Effective care for high need patients: opportunities for improving outcomes, value, and health. National Academy of Medicine. 2017

One of the core responsibilities of PACE is to provide continuity of care across settings to achieve improved patient outcomes and reduce complications. Because of integrated interdisciplinary team involvement, complications such as medication errors and potentially avoidable hospitalizations are reduced because of this proactive care. PACE programs have 16% lower 30-day all cause hospital readmission rates compared to all dual-eligible Medicare beneficiaries 65 years and older. Recent data also indicates a 24% lower hospitalization rate in PACE participants compared to dual-eligible nursing home residents on Medicaid. The PACE model of care is successful because there are direct and frequent interactions between the participants and their interdisciplinary team which allows the flexibility to customize services to each participant and adapt quickly to changes in their health.

Case Example

Kathy is a 74-year old woman who lives independently in her own apartment. She has several chronic medical conditions including poorly controlled diabetes, atrial fibrillation, and congestive heart failure with reduced ejection fraction. In addition, she has multiple chemical sensitivities, which makes being out of her apartment very challenging to her as she has reactions to many commonly used chemicals. On enrollment in her local PACE organization, she expressed a desire to avoid hospitalization if possible. She often falls in the middle of the night and must call 9-1-1 to help her get off the floor. Medics have noted very elevated blood sugars on arrival to her home.

The PACE team discusses her often during their regular interdisciplinary team meetings and works hard to support her in the home. The PT and OT make home visits to assess her home safety, making suggestions to clear the clutter in her apartment and get her appropriate adaptive equipment including a four wheeled walker.

The PCP, RN CM, and RD work together on her diabetes control – discussing appropriate foods for her as well as educating and monitoring for medication compliance. The team feels that she would not be able to handle self-administration of insulin in her current home setting, and therefore she is managed with oral medications which are closely monitored by the IDT.

PACE programs are well suited to take a pro-active role in keeping patients out of the hospital. **Through IDT involvement with biannual assessment and discussion at care plan meetings and regular follow up, subtle changes can be identified early and acted upon**. All members of the care team, including van drivers, healthcare aides, caregivers at facilities, and PACE center staff are involved in monitoring PACE participants. If a change in condition is noted and shared with the IDT, that participant can be quickly assessed, and a plan of care put into place in response to this change in status. Members of the participant's IDT are a phone call away and can be recruited to help with assessment and management.

In addition, the creation and maintenance of a personalized and updated care plan allows PACE IDT members to be aware of a participant's baseline level of cognitive and physical function as well as goals of care. Providing necessary medical equipment and supplies, medication, nutritional support, home care services and transportation to follow up appointments can help keep PACE participants safe and well supported in their home setting and avoid hospitalization related to a change in condition. In addition, ongoing conversations about goals of care and meaningful advance care planning with family and/or designated decision makers can assist in determining whether or not hospitalization is consistent with a participant's goals.

Despite the PACE IDT's involvement in getting her home setting less cluttered, sending appropriate adaptive equipment out to the home, and providing education on diabetes management, Kathy has a fall at home and is unable to bear weight on her leg. The nurse case manager visits her at home, discusses options and they both decide she should go to the hospital given her uncontrolled pain and inability to care for herself. Consideration was given to putting her in a SNF to avoid hospitalization, but ultimately the PCP and RN CM decide that an ER visit would likely expedite workup and possible treatment. In the ER she is noted to have a hip fracture, and she is hospitalized with a plan for operative repair.

PACE programs provide coordination across settings. Because of the focus on providing the right care at the right time, PACE providers are comfortable with managing the risks associated with caring for a population of frail older adults in the community and are often more knowledgeable about resources to support that participant. Without the involvement of a PACE PCP, there is a high likelihood that a frail, medically complex PACE participant who ends up in a hospital emergency department will be admitted. Communication between the PACE PCP or RN case manager and the emergency room providers helps to determine if a patient truly needs hospitalization or if other supports can be put into place to allow that person to discharge to a less acute care setting. Because PACE organizations coordinate all care, extra home care may be arranged or a brief stay in a SNF to stabilize the patient before returning home. **Because of the payment structure, PACE organizations are able to utilize the SNF benefit without a qualifying hospital stay**.

If a patient is considered unstable and a decision is made to hospitalize that person, then the PACE interdisciplinary team is actively involved from day 1 of hospitalization in coordinating with the inpatient team and the discharge planner at the hospital. PACE staff are able to provide helpful information on prior level of physical and cognitive function, as well as the level of care that can be provided in the patient's current home setting. This allows the inpatient team to help determine whether a higher level of care is needed to allow for recovery prior to returning to their home setting. If a participant is readmitted or has recurrent hospitalizations, PACE programs look at utilization and work to problem solve, determining the underlying causes of readmission, and whether any supports can be put into place to prevent this from happening again.

Kathy is in the hospital for about a week. Her hip fracture is repaired uneventfully but she has some post-operative heart failure which requires adjustment in her diuretics. The hospital team also decides to start her on insulin given significant elevation in blood sugars and concern for optimizing healing from her surgery. The PACE IDT in consultation with the hospitalist team decide that she needs extra time to recuperate in a SNF before consideration can be given to her returning home.

If a hospitalized PACE participant experiences a decline in functional or cognitive status, home support offered by the PACE organization (such as extra home care hours or increase in PT or OT visits) might not be sufficient to ensure safety at home. In such circumstances, PACE programs can utilize skilled nursing facilities (SNF) to provide rehabilitative care. Because of the continuity of care across settings, PACE teams can ensure that the care plan determined during hospitalization is carried out and medications appropriately reconciled. Throughout the participant's stay in the SNF, the PACE IDT continues to collaborate with the SNF care team: there is no "hand off" of care responsibility to the SNF. Each PACE discipline maintains communication with their equivalent discipline in the SNF—the PT and OT team communicate with the SNF rehab team to discuss prior level of function and equipment needs, the RD communicates dietary care plan changes, the MSW works with the social worker at the SNF to ensure a safe discharge, and PCPs provide ongoing medical visits and coordination of specialty appointments and follow up. This allows continuation of the care plan determined in the hospital for ongoing recovery of the acute health condition as well as quick follow up and care coordination.

Kathy makes good progress in the SNF, ambulating with a four wheeled walker. After discussions with Kathy and her DPOA, the team decides that she would benefit from a care setting with a higher level of support where she can receive help with her diabetes and CHF management as well as give her some assistance with ADLs. The team is able to find an assisted living facility (ALF) which offers supportive care which meet her current needs. She thrives at the ALF: surprisingly, her multiple chemical sensitivity syndrome is not as bothersome, she is able to socialize with others, have meals prepared for her and even takes on the task of organizing the ALF's library.

PACE programs are equipped to determine safety in the home setting. Occupational therapists provide home safety assessments at the time of enrollment and adaptive equipment is put into place to allow participants to function as safely as possible. Dieticians optimize nutrition by taking detailed dietary histories and providing supplementation if nutritional needs are not met. The **social worker makes sure decision makers are identified and behavioral health supports are in place**. If, despite all of the supports that the PACE program offers, care needs cannot be met in the prior living situation, the PACE IDT can work with contracted facilities to find the appropriate location where adequate support can be given. This often helps alleviate family and caregiver burden, as it can be overwhelming to find a new place for a frail and medically complex older adult to move. Transition to the new setting is also eased by the knowledge of the PACE team who can provide support and education to the new caregivers about the individual participant. Respite can be provided by attendance at day health centers while the participant adjusts to their new setting. Medication reconciliation is again completed as a participant moves from one location to another. Care planning is completed by the team and shared with the providers at the ALF to provide consistency in care.

Kathy does well at the ALF for a year. Initially because she was doing well, her goals of care change and she desires more interventions than when she enrolled in the PACE organization. Over the ensuing months, she has a couple of hospitalizations for heart failure and chest pain. Fortunately, these are brief (2-3 days each) due to the frequent communication and coordination between the hospital care team and the PACE care team. After her second hospitalization, she decides she does not want to go to the hospital any longer. Plans are made to enroll her in the comfort care program (Hospice equivalent) to provide support for her to help her remain in the home setting.

Care at the end-of-life outside of the PACE model is often fragmented and poorly coordinated among different health providers. These transitions can be burdensome to older adults as well as their families and caregivers. **Ongoing and active advance care planning and conversations regarding participant goals of care and values helps the PACE IDT support a participant in determining what matters most to them**. This helps align the care plan with the participant goals of care and allows the team to take a proactive role in end-of-life support and planning. Evidence suggests that regular discussions and documentation of advanced care planning can lead to less-aggressive care at the end of life because it allows more time to weave knowledge of patient preferences with the plan for their care. Many PACE programs provide Hospice-level services or contract with Hospice programs to help support participants in remaining comfortable through end-of-life and avoiding unnecessary hospitalizations at the end-of-life.

Summary

PACE organizations, by virtue of active involvement of the interdisciplinary team and proactive care planning and assessment, are well-equipped to provide thorough care coordination across the various settings in which their PACE participants receive care. Because of this, transitions of care are smoother and less fraught with challenges including re-hospitalization, medication errors, duplication of care, or unmet needs. Because of the unique model, PACE organizations have been able to demonstrate reduced hospitalization and re-admission rates, lower lengths of stay in hospitals, and improved care at the end-of-life.

Suggested Reading

Naylor MD, Aiken LH, Kurtzman ET, Olds DM, Hirschman KB. The importance of transitional care in achieving health reform. Health Aff. 2011;30(4) https://doi.org/10.1377/HLTHAFF.2011.0041.

Long P, et al. Effective care for high need patients: opportunities for improving outcomes, value, and health. Washington, DC: National Academy of Medicine; 2017. https://nam.edu/wp-content/uploads/2017/06/Effective-Care-for-High-Need-Patients.pdf

Finlayson K, et al. Transitional care interventions reduce unplanned hospital readmissions in high-risk older adults. BMC Health Serv Res. 2018;18(1):956. https://doi.org/10.1186/s12913-018-3771-9.

Gyurmey T, Kwiatkowski J. Program of all-inclusive care for the elderly (PACE): integrating health and social care since 1973. RI Med J. 2019;102(5):30–2.

Programs of All-Inclusive Care for the Elderly (PACE) Manual. https://www.cms.gov/Regulations-and-Guidance/Guidance/Manuals/Internet-Only-Manuals-IOMs-Items/CMS019036. Accessed 13 Jul 2020.

Segelman M, Szydlowski J, Kinosian B, McNabney M, Raziano D, Eng C, van Reenen C, Temkin-Greener H. Hospitalizations in the program of all-inclusive care for the elderly. J Am Geriatr Soc. 2014;62:320–4. https://doi.org/10.1111/jgs.12637.

Meret-Hanke L. Effects of the program of all-inclusive care for the elderly on hospital use. Gerontologist. 2011;51(6):774–85. https://doi.org/10.1093/geront/gnr040.

Coleman E. Falling through the cracks: challenges and opportunities for improving transitional care for persons with continuous complex care needs. J Am Geriatr Soc. 2003;51(4):549–55. https://doi.org/10.1046/j.1532-5415.2003.51185.

Gleckman H. Coordinating care: an elusive but critical goal. In: Health progress; 2009. p. 32–5.

Pak E, Perfetto C, Yu Q, McNabney M. Effect of enrollment in the program of all-inclusive care for the elderly on end-of-life care. J Am Geriatr Soc. 2012;60(1):166–7. https://doi.org/10.1111/j.1532-5415.2011.03745.x.

Patel E, McNabney M. Evaluation of emergency room visits and subsequent hospitalization within the programs of all-inclusive care for the elderly. Geriatr Gerontol Int. 2020;20(5):503–5. https://doi.org/10.1111/ggi.13899.

National PACE Association: PACE by the numbers. 2020. https://www.npaonline.org/sites/default/files/3186_pace_infographic_update_121819_combined_v1.pdf. Accessed 10 Jul 2020.

PACE Medical Directors Handbook: https://www.npaonline.org/pace-medical-directors-handbook.

Sarnak D, Ryan J. How high-need patients experience the health care system in nine countries. New York: The Commonwealth Fund; 2016. https://www.commonwealthfund.org/publications/issue-briefs/2016/jan/how-high-need-patients-experience-health-care-system-nine. Accessed 20 Jul 2020.

Segelman M, Szydlowski J, Kinosian B, McNabney M, Raziano D, Eng C, van Reenen C, Temkin-Greener H. Hospitalizations in the program of all-inclusive Care for the Elderly. J Am Geriatr Soc. 2014;62(2):320–4. https://doi.org/10.1111/jgs.12637.

The Care Transitions Program. https://caretransitions.org/about-the-care-transitions-intervention/. Accessed 19 Apr 2021.

Continuity of Care: The Transitional Care Model. http://ojin.nursingworld.org/MainMenuCategories/ANAMarketplace/ANAPeriodicals/OJIN/TableofContents/Vol-20-2015/No3-Sept-2015/Continuity-of-Care-Transitional-Care-Model.html#:~:text=The%20Transitional%20Care%20Model%20(TCM),-The%20TCM%20supplements&text=The%20TCM%20intervention%20focuses%20on,centered%20medical%20homes%20(PCMHs). Accessed 19 Apr 2021.

Chapter 23
End-of-Life Care in PACE

David Wensel

End-of-life care in the United States continues to be very complicated and fractured. Congress created a permanent provision to Medicare including the Hospice Benefit in 1986, after studying the provision for more than 10 years. It was determined that the benefit should be available to anyone who qualifies for Medicare and has about 6 months or less to live. The key word being "about" since very few medical providers are accurate at predicting how long someone will live. This leads to the problem of so many people enrolling in their Medicare Hospice Benefit very late in their disease process. Many Medicare beneficiaries receive Hospice care for less than 14 days, although they could benefit from this care for many months.

This causes some real difficulties for patients and their families. Often when patients enroll in the Medicare Hospice Benefit, it is after a long hospital stay with or without a skilled nursing facility admission. Most Medicare beneficiaries have a Primary Care Provider that they see in clinic usually every few months. When they have a medical event that lands them in the hospital, it is usually related to some significant physical decline. They are cared for in the hospital by a completely different medical team and different physicians. If they are discharged to a skilled nursing facility, they are often cared for by yet another completely different medical team and another physician. When patients do enroll in the Medicare Hospice Benefit, they are cared for by the Hospice team, which includes a nurse, social worker, chaplain, physical therapist, volunteer coordinator, bereavement coordinator and the Hospice Medical Director. Most Primary Care Physicians do not have time to manage their patients who are enrolled in the Medicare Hospice Benefit, especially when the patients can no longer travel into the office for visits. This leads to fragmented care that does not always align with the values and goals of the patient and their caregivers.

D. Wensel (✉)
TRU Community Care, Lafayette, CO, USA
e-mail: davidwensel@trucare.org

M. K. McNabney (ed.), *Community-Based Integrated Care for Older Adults*,
https://doi.org/10.1007/978-3-031-05137-1_23

Palliative Medicine is specialized medical care for people living with a serious illness and suffering. This type of care is focused on providing relief from the symptoms and stress of illness. The goal is to improve quality of life for both the patient and the family when patients have more than 6 months to live. This allows for a medical team of specialist to follow patients over a longer period for their care. This is primarily provided by a Physician, Advanced Practice Registered Nurse, Social Worker, and possibly a Chaplain. The Palliative Medicine Interdisciplinary Team (IDT) is much smaller than the PACE IDT, or the Medicare Hospice Benefit IDT.

PACE (Program of All-Inclusive Care of the Elderly) is a Medicare and Medicaid certified program that has all the elements of quality Palliative Medicine and Hospice Care. This includes an IDT of Physicians, Advanced Practice Registered Nurse, Registered Nurse, Social Workers, Physical Therapist, Occupational Therapist, Transportation, Dietician, Home Health Aides, Life Enrichment specialist, Chaplains, and Bereavement services. This provides for a person-centered approach to care with a comprehensive care plan that meets the needs of participants, supports the family, and caregivers. **PACE is able to develop a long-term relationship with the participant and their caregivers**. This serves to ensure that the care provided to them aligns with their values and goals.

PACE serves very frail elderly people who are 55 years of age or older, and nursing home eligible with a limited life expectancy. This frailty is often due to multiple chronic medical conditions along with physical and cognitive decline. Most PACE participants depend on assistance with at least two of their Activities of Daily Living (ADL). They require a lot of care to remain living safely in the community that is coordinated, and often provided, by an IDT. Since most PACE participants struggle with life limiting illness and physical symptoms, they would be appropriate for Palliative Medicine consultation. PACE is able to provide the care needed to address suffering and support PACE participants, especially as they decline.

Medicare requires that PACE organizations provide all the usual care that anyone who is not enrolled in PACE would receive under their Medicare Benefit. **PACE participants usually have a prolonged, gradual decline in function leading up to their death. PACE participants have an average life expectancy of around 34 months from the time they enroll, remaining in PACE throughout their decline**. PACE organizations have an opportunity to meet the needs of these participants by using the IDT to develop a Care Plan that is individualized to the needs of each PACE participant. By caring for this population over a longer period of time, the care can be tailored to meet the specific needs of PACE participants and their families.

In the PACE model of care, the IDT can provide care that will relieve suffering and support family and caregivers long before PACE participants would be eligible to receive this type of care under the usual Medicare Model. The major benefit of this for participants is the primary medical team does not change regardless of care setting. PACE organizations are expected to continue providing high quality care to PACE participants throughout their physical decline including hospitalization, facility placement, and end-of-life care. The PACE team builds a supportive relationship with participants, caregivers, and their families over time. This allows the care that is provided to address any suffering and improve the quality of life for the participants.

Medicare and Medicaid will not allow a PACE participant to enroll in the Medicare Hospice Benefit while being enrolled in PACE. That is seen as double payment for the same services. PACE organizations provide all the core services of the Medicare Hospice Benefit by utilizing the IDT, which typically has more members than the Hospice IDT. This allows the participant to remain living independently in the community longer with the support of the PACE IDT. When frail older adults are allowed to live longer and safely in the community, they report the quality of their life as better. With the care being provided by the same IDT throughout the disease trajectory, the participants are more likely to allow help in their homes.

Because the life expectancy of a PACE participant is longer than 6 months when they enroll in PACE, the IDT can form a close relationship with the participant and their families to provide better coordinated care. The PACE IDT works to align that care with the values, goals, and wishes of each PACE participant. The core members of the PACE IDT can quickly address any suffering they recognize due to this closer relationship. The PACE IDT is also able to support family and caregivers over a longer period of time as the participant declines. The IDT members can discuss ongoing issues with caregivers and family as they become aware of them. This preparation can serve to provide opportunity for anticipatory grieving to take place, long before the PACE participants die.

There is more value in supporting PACE participants that are cared for by a familiar team who understands their values, needs, and wishes. This continuity of care provided by the PACE IDT allows participants to remain at home and get the care they need, when they need it. The PACE participants, caregivers, and family members can become more familiar with the IDT members and develop a stronger sense of trust with the care that is provided.

There are three basic ways a PACE organization can provide Palliative Medicine and End-of-Life Care. The first approach is to provide all the care that is needed by the PACE IDT members as it is needed. This can be done when the PACE IDT members feel comfortable with the skills of providing this care. Good Palliative Medicine and End-of-Life care is a skill set that can be developed in any PACE IDT. It usually requires at least one champion on the PACE IDT who has interest in learning more about this and teaching others. The **second approach is for a PACE organization to partner with a local Palliative Medicine and Hospice team to help with providing this care**. This is an excellent way to get the PACE IDT members more experience and training when working with experts who provide the care. This collaborative approach allows the care to continue being provided by familiar PACE IDT members, while introducing a small number of new team members from a Hospice and Palliative Medicine program. The **final approach is to allow the PACE participant to enroll in their Medicare Hospice Benefit, which will automatically disenroll them from the PACE program**. This last approach is the most disruptive for the PACE participant by replacing the IDT members with a new group.

Also notice the use of the phrase "End-of-Life" care rather than Hospice. This is intentional since Hospice is a defined Medicare Benefit and in a PACE program it is provided the care when it is needed. All PACE participants deserve excellent Palliative Medicine and End-of-Life care no matter how the PACE organization decides to provide it. This care should always be aligned with the values and goals of the PACE participant, their families and caregivers. When PACE provides the care needed, including End-of-Life care, the PACE organization can follow the family and caregivers for bereavement support as well. Many PACE organizations are providing this support with existing IDT members or partnering with local resources to provide the support.

It is very important to acknowledge the support which is needed by the PACE IDT members themselves, as they care for frail participant who die. Caring for these people over time and supporting them to die with comfort and dignity is often difficult emotionally for the PACE IDT. It is always helpful to support the PACE IDT members by allowing them to grieve as well. Unlike the usual Medicare Primary Care model that will be notified when a person they care for dies. Most of the PACE IDT members are providing the care needed in the home of participants as they decline, need more support, and aware when they die.

Summary

PACE organizations have a great opportunity and responsibility to provide care to some of the frailest individuals and their families. This allows the PACE IDT to impact the way that care is given, making sure it always matches the values, goals, and wishes of those we serve.

Suggested Reading

Eng C. Future considerations for improving end-of-life care for older persons: program of all-inclusive care for the elderly. J Palliat Med. 2002;5:305–10.

Hughes MT, Smith TJ. The growth of palliative care in the United States. Annu Rev Public Health. 2014;35:459–75.

Morton C, Prichett L, McNabney M. Opioid prescriptions and health care utilization at end of life in a program of all-inclusive care for the elderly. J Am Med Dir Assoc. 2020;221:1362–3.

Pak E, Perfetto C, Yu Q, McNabney M. Effect of enrollment in the program of all-inclusive care for the elderly on end-of-life care. J Am Geriatr Soc. 2012;60:166–7.

Temkin-Greener H, Mukamel DB. Predicting place of death in the program of all-inclusive care for the elderly: participant versus program characteristics. J Am Geriatr Soc. 2002;50:125–35.

Index

M. K. McNabney (ed.), *Community-Based Integrated Care for Older Adults*, https://doi.org/10.1007/978-3-031-05137-1

E

F

G

H

I

MIX
Papier aus verantwortungsvollen Quellen
Paper from responsible sources
FSC® C105338

If you have any concerns about our products,
you can contact us on
ProductSafety@springernature.com

In case Publisher is established outside the EU,
the EU authorized representative is:
Springer Nature Customer Service Center GmbH
Europaplatz 3, 69115 Heidelberg, Germany

Printed by Libri Plureos GmbH
in Hamburg, Germany